How to
GRILL
EVERYTHING

THE ULTIMATE DELICIOUS, FLAVORFUL RECIPES
PLUS TIPS AND TRICKS FOR BEGINNERS
AND ADVANCED PITMASTERS.

GRAHAM K. WILSON

W0008241

Table of Contents

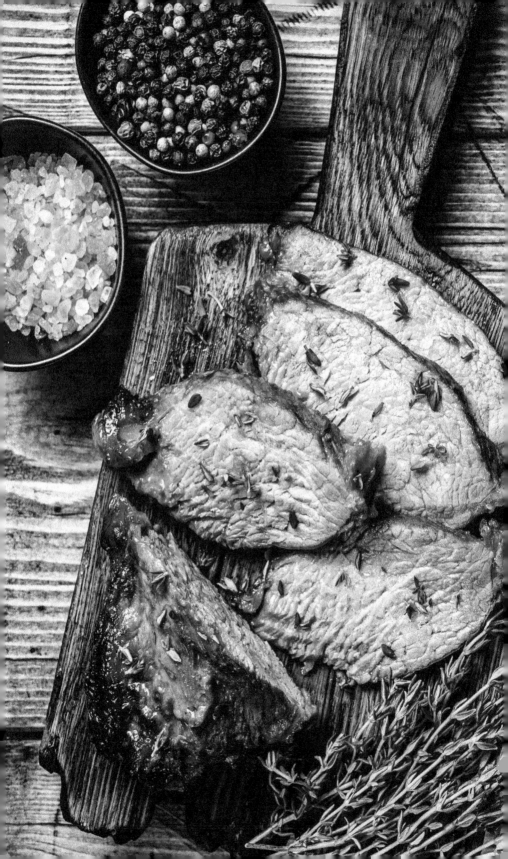

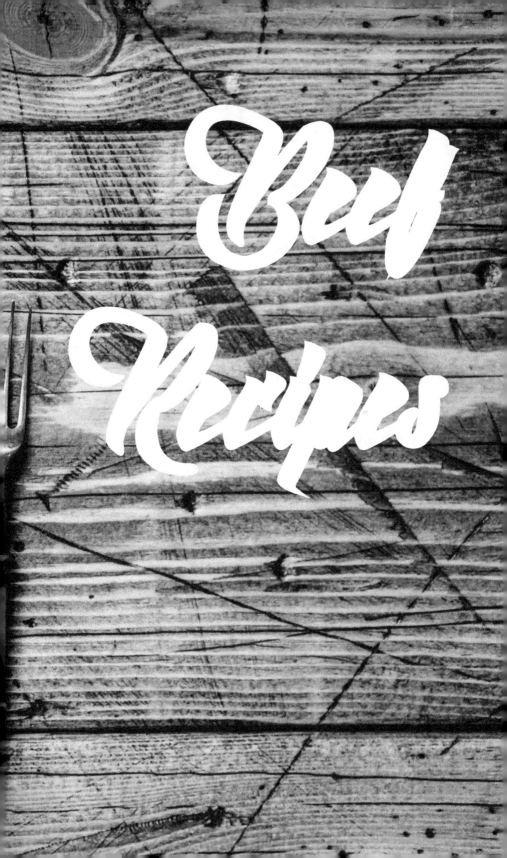

Beef Recipes

BETTER THAN SEX
T-BONE STEAKS

Prep. Time: 10 min	Cook Time: 8 min	Servings: 8

NUTRITION

Calories: 897 | Fat: 41g |Carbs: 2.8g | Protein: 119g.

INGREDIENTS

- 8 T-bone steaks at room temperature (16 ounce)
- 2 tbsp. salt, or to taste
- 1 tbsp. black pepper
- 2 tsp. onion powder.
- 1 tbsp. paprika.
- 2 tsp. ground turmeric, or to taste
- 2 tsp. ground coriander, or to taste
- 2 tsp. garlic powder, or to taste.
- 2 tsp. cayenne pepper, or to taste.

DIRECTIONS

1. Preheat an outdoor grill for high heat, and lightly oil the grate.

2. In a small bowl, mix the black pepper, salt, garlic powder onion powder, coriander, cayenne pepper, turmeric and paprika; set aside.

3. Rub the steaks on all sides with the seasoning mixture

4. Cook on the preheated grill to your desired degree of doneness, about 3 minutes per side for medium-rare.

5. The ideal temperature is 130°F.

6. Your amazing T-Bone steaks are ready!

AMAZING BBQ STEAK

Prep. Time: 20 min	Cook Time: 16 min	Servings: 9

NUTRITION

Calories: 427 | Fats: 32g | Carbs: 4.9g | Protein: 26g.

INGREDIENTS

- 1½ tri-tip steak (2 ounce)
- 1½ small onion, chopped
- ¾ cup olive oil
- ¾ cup vinegar
- 10½ cloves garlic
- 3 tbsp. prepared mustard
- 3 tbsp. chopped fresh rosemary
- ¾ cup soy sauce
- 1 tsp. black pepper
- 1 tsp. of magic shrimp seasoning.
- 1 tbsp. salt

DIRECTIONS

1. Put olive oil, garlic, onion, soy sauce, vinegar, rosemary, salt, mustard, and pepper into the bowl of a food processor.

2. Process until smooth.

3. Put steak in a large resealable plastic bag.

4. Pour marinade over steaks, seal, then refrigerate for about 2 hours 45 minutes.

5. Preheat the grill for high heat.

6. Brush grill grate with oil. Discard marinade, and place steak on the prepared grill.

7. Cook for about 8 minutes per side.

TASTY CHATEAUBRIAND

| Prep. Time: 1 hour | Cook Time: 10 min | Servings: 4 |

NUTRITION

Calories: 697 | Fats: 49g | Carbs: 4g | Protein: 59g.

INGREDIENTS

- 4 beef tenderloin filets (1 1/2 inch thick)
- Ground black pepper to taste
- ¼ cup butter
- ¼ cup vegetable oil

DIRECTIONS

1. Rub the beef with the vegetable oil and season with freshly ground black pepper.

2. Let the beef rest at room temperature for about 50/55 minutes.

3. Heat a large, heavy skillet over medium-high heat. Quickly sear the meat about 6/7 seconds on each side, then remove from skillet.

4. Melt and gild the butter in the skillet.

5. Return the meat to the skillet, and fry 4 to 5 minutes on each side.

6. Remove from the skillet and let stand for about 6/7 minutes for the juices to settle. Enjoy!

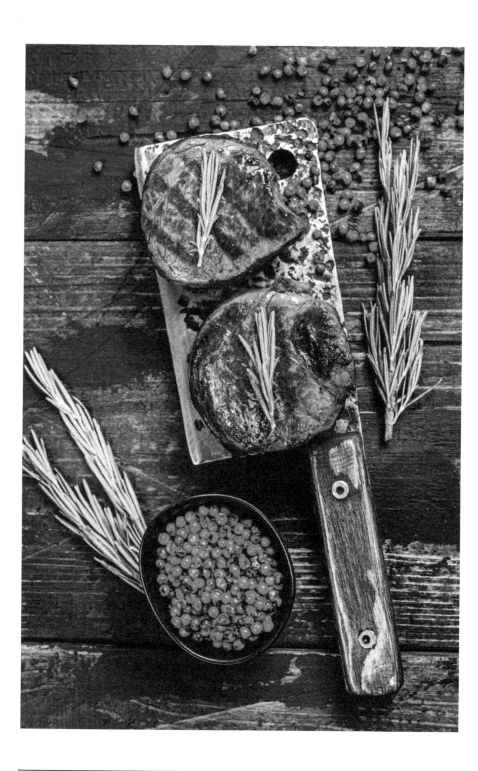

PERFECT FILET MIGNONS

Prep. Time: 15 min   Cook Time: 18 min   Servings: 8

NUTRITION

Calories: 539 | Fats: 43g | Carbs: 5g | Protein: 31g.

INGREDIENTS

- 8 filet mignon steaks (1 1/2 inch thick)
- ½ cup coarsely crushed black peppercorns
- 2 tbsp. butter
- Salt, to taste
- ⅔ cup beef broth
- 2 tsp. olive oil
- 2 cups heavy cream

DIRECTIONS

1. Put the peppercorns into a small bowl.

2. Sprinkle the beef tenderloin filets with salt on both sides, and coat both sides with crushed peppercorns.

3. Melt the butter with the olive oil over high heat in a heavy skillet (not nonstick) until the foam disappears from the butter.

4. Put the steaks in the pan.

5. Cook until they start to become pink/red and juicy in the center, about 3 minutes per side

6. An instant-read thermometer inserted into the center should read 125°F.

7. Remove the steaks to platter and cover tightly with foil.

8. Pour the beef broth into the skillet, and use a whip to mix the broth

9. Blend the cream, and simmer the sauce until it's thickened and reduced, 7 to 8 minutes

10. Place the steaks back in the skillet, turn to coat with sauce

11. Serve with the remaining sauce over.

MEDITERRANEAN RIBEYE

| Prep. Time: 20 min | Cook Time: 15 min | Servings: 6 |

NUTRITION

Calories: 387 | Fats: 31g | Carbs: 6g | Protein: 29g

INGREDIENTS

- 6 boneless beef ribeye steaks, cut 1 inch thick
- 2 tbsp. fresh oregano, chopped
- 18 garlic cloves, roughly chopped
- 2 tsp. pepper
- 2 tbsp. chopped fresh parsley
- 2 tbsp. chopped fresh basil
- 2 tbsp. kosher salt
- 2 tsp. chopped fresh rosemary
- ¼ cup balsamic vinegar
- 1 cup olive oil

DIRECTIONS

1. Put the oregano, basil, garlic, parsley, salt and rosemary, into a small bowl, and mash into a coarse paste.

2. Mix in the olive oil, pepper and balsamic vinegar until blended.

3. Take half of the mixture and put it into a separate small bowl; set aside.

4. Spread the remaining half of the herb mixture evenly over the steaks. Set aside to marinate for 50/55 minutes.

5. Preheat an outdoor grill for medium-high heat, and lightly oil the grate.

6. Cook the steaks on the preheated grill for about 8 minutes, then turn over, and coat with the herb mixture.

7. Cook for other about 8 minutes more for medium-well, or until your favorite degree of doneness has been reached.

YUMMY JUICY STEAKS

NUTRITION

Calories: 367 | Fats: 27g | Carbs: 7g | Protein: 21g

INGREDIENTS

- 8 rib-eye steaks
- ½ cup canola oil
- ½ cup root beer
- 1 tsp. dried rosemary
- ¼ cup Worcestershire sauce
- 1 tsp. ground thyme
- ¼ cup steak sauce
- ¼ cup teriyaki sauce
- 1 tsp. ground black pepper
- 1 tsp. onion salt
- 2 tsp. garlic salt
- 1 tsp. onion salt.

DIRECTIONS

1. In a bowl mix together the root beer, canola oil, teriyaki sauce, Worcestershire sauce, garlic salt, steak sauce, black pepper, basil, onion salt, rosemary and thyme.

2. Pierce the steaks on both sides; arrange in a single layer in a shallow dish. Pour the marinade over the steaks, flipping the meat to coat both sides.

3. Allow to marinate in refrigerator 3 hours and a half, flipping meat once halfway through.

4. Preheat an outdoor grill for medium-high heat, and lightly oil the grate.

5. Remove the steaks from the marinade, then discard the remaining marinade.

6. Cook the steaks until they are beginning to firm, and are hot and slightly pink in the center, about 6 minutes per side.

7. The ideal temperature is 135°F for medium.

AMAZING LONDON BROIL

Prep. Time: 35 min   Cook Time: 20 min   Servings: 4

NUTRITION

Calories: 183 | Fat: 11g | Carbs: 1g | Protein: 27g.

INGREDIENTS

- 2 lb. flank steak
- ½ clove garlic, minced
- ¼ tsp. dried oregano
- ½ tsp. salt
- 2 tbsp. soy sauce
- 1 tbsp. ketchup
- ½ tsp. black pepper
- ½ tsp. vegetable oil

DIRECTIONS

1. In a bowl, mix together salt, garlic, ketchup, soy sauce, black pepper, vegetable oil, and oregano.

2. Score both sides of the meat with a fork. Rub garlic mixture into both sides of the meat.

3. Wrap tightly in aluminum foil, and refrigerate for 4 to 5 hours, or for all the night. Flip meat every few hours.

4. Preheat an outdoor grill for high heat, and lightly oil grate.

5. Place meat on the prepared grill. Cook for 4 to 6 minutes per side, or to reach your favorite cooking.

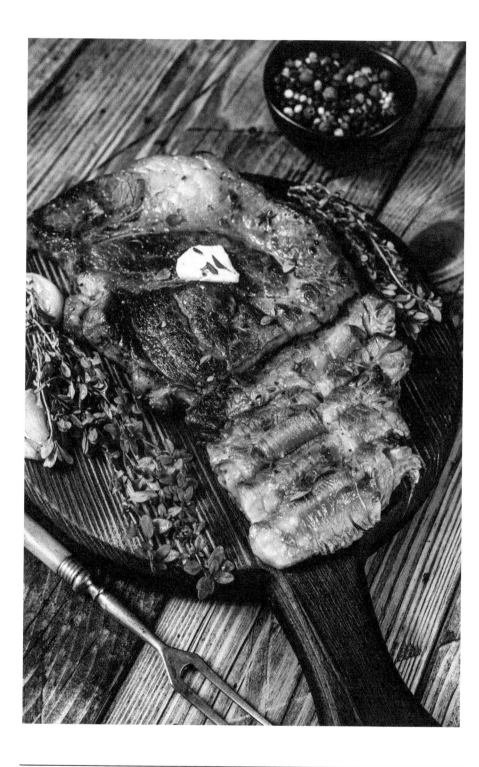

"WOW EFFECT" STEAK MARINADE

Prep. Time: 15 min	Cook Time: 20 min	Servings: 4

NUTRITION

Calories: 683 | Fat: 49g | Carbs: 25g | Protein: 31g.

INGREDIENTS

- 4 boneless rib-eye steaks
- 1 tsp garlic powder, or to taste
- Salt, to taste
- Black pepper, to taste
- Steak seasoning, to taste

Marinade

- 6 cloves garlic, chopped
- ⅔ cup extra virgin olive oil
- ⅔ cup soy sauce
- ⅔ cup balsamic vinegar
- ⅔ cup Worcestershire sauce
- ⅓ cup mustard

DIRECTIONS

1. Put steaks in a container.

2. Cut slits in the fat around the edges of the steaks. Gently pierce both sides of each steak a few times with a fork.

3. Sprinkle each steak with garlic powder, pepper, salt, and steak seasoning.

4. Spread seasonings into steaks.

5. In a bowl, mix together Worcestershire sauce, soy sauce, olive oil, mustard, garlic and balsamic vinegar.

6. Pour marinade over steaks to coat.

7. Cover container with plastic wrap and marinate steaks in the refrigerator for a couple of hours.

8. Turn steaks over and marinate for another couple of hours.

9. Preheat an outdoor grill for medium-high heat and lightly oil the grate.

10. Cook the steaks on the preheated grill until they start to be reddish-pink and juicy in the center, 7 to 9

minutes per side for medium-rare (ideal temperature should be 125°F).

Tip: you can leave the steaks in your marinade for 6 hours, or better 12 hours.

NOT AN ORDINARY STEAK

NUTRITION

Calories: 339 | Total Fat: 194g | Carbs: 14g | Protein: 26g.

INGREDIENTS

- 4 lb. cubed beef stew meat
- ⅔ cup corn syrup
- ½ cup soy sauce
- 2 tsp. minced garlic
- 2 tsp. salt
- 1 tbsp. Greek seasoning, or to taste

DIRECTIONS

1. In a large bow, mix the corn syrup, garlic, salt and soy sauce.

2. Season the meat with Greek seasoning

3. Add the beef and marinate for up to 20 hours, flipping over few times to evenly marinate.

4. Preheat a grill for medium heat. When hot, lightly oil the grate. Then, thread the beef cubes onto skewers

5. Grill the meat on the preheated grill, turning occasionally, until they have reached your favorite doneness.

6. Don't worry if steak become dark, it's because of syrup sugar. Enjoy!

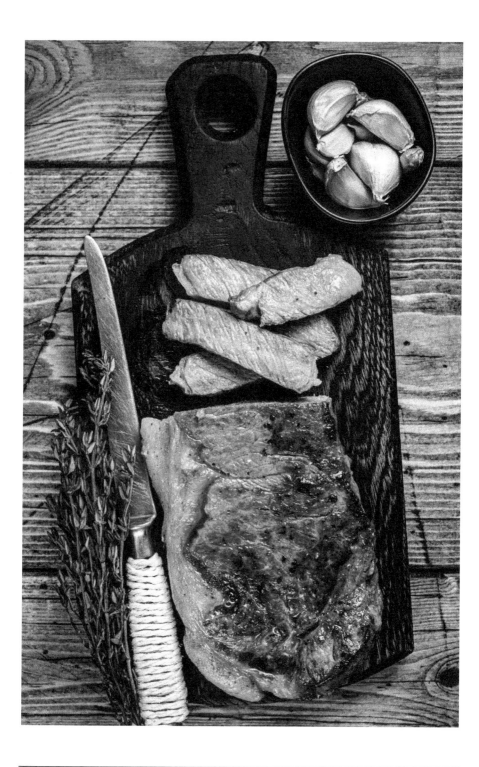

NY BBQ STEAK

Prep. Time: 25 min   Cook Time: 30 min   Servings: 8

NUTRITION

Calories: 177 | Fat: 8g | Protein: 22g | Carbs: 3g.

INGREDIENTS

- 8 beef strip steaks (1¼-inch-thick)
- 1 tbsp. finely chopped garlic
- 4 tbsp. olive oil
- ½ cup salted butter
- 1 tbsp. salt
- 2 tsp. black pepper
- 6 sage sprigs
- 10 rosemary sprigs
- 10 thyme sprigs

DIRECTIONS

1. Preheat grill to high (460°F to 540°F).

2. Put steaks on a baking sheet, drizzle with olive oil, and sprinkle with salt and pepper.

3. Let stand, covered, at room temperature about 25 minutes.

4. Meanwhile, gather thyme, sage sprigs and rosemary, in a tight bundle, and tie stem ends with kitchen twine.

5. Melt butter in a small skillet over medium-low. Add garlic, and cook, mixing often, about 1 minute. Then, remove from heat.

6. Place steaks on oiled grates, and grill, uncovered, a couple of minutes.

7. Turn steaks 45° to create diagonal grill marks. Grill, uncovered, until grill marks appear, about 2-3 minutes.

8. Turn steaks over, and grill, uncovered, until a thermometer registers 145°F when inserted in thickest portion of steak, about 6 minutes.

9. Brush steaks often with garlic butter, using herb bundle as a brush.

10. Transfer steaks to a cutting board and let rest 7 to 9 minutes before slicing.

11. Discard herb bundle and serve. Enjoy!

GRILLED STEAK DINNER TONIGHT!

Prep. Time: 25 min   Cook Time: 15 min   Servings: 4

NUTRITION

Calories: 437 | Protein: 27g | Carbs: 3g | Fat: 33g.

INGREDIENTS

- 4 tbsp. olive oil
- 2 tsp. steak seasoning
- 2 tbsp. butter, melted
- 2 tbsp. white wine
- 4 filets mignon steaks
- 2 tbsp. finely minced onion
- 2 tbsp. Worcestershire sauce
- 24 medium shrimp, peeled and deveined
- 2 tsp. lemon juice
- ¼ tsp. ground black pepper
- 2 clove garlic, minced
- 2 tsp. dried parsley
- 2 tsp. seafood seasoning

DIRECTIONS

1. Mix 1 tbsp. butter, olive oil, wine, onion, garlic, Worcestershire sauce, parsley, lemon juice, seafood seasoning, and black pepper together in a bowl; then add shrimp. Mix to coat evenly.

2. Cover bowl with plastic wrap and refrigerate for flavors to blend, at least 15/20 minutes.

3. Preheat an outdoor grill for medium-high heat and lightly oil the grate.

4. Coat steaks with 1 tbsp. olive oil; sprinkle with steak seasoning.

5. Cook steaks until they are beginning to firm and have reached your favorite doneness, about 6 minutes per side. An instant-read thermometer inserted into the center should read 145 °F.

6. Transfer steaks to a platter and loosely tent with a piece of aluminum foil.

7. Remove shrimp from marinade and grill until they are bright pink on the outside, a couple of minutes per side.

ORIGINAL SIRLOIN KABOBS

Prep. Time: 20 min	Cook Time: 20 min	Servings: 4

NUTRITION

Calories: 319 | Fat: 15g | Carbs: 17g | Protein: 25g.

INGREDIENTS

- 1 lb. beef sirloin steak, cut into 1 inch cubes
- Skewers
- 2 tbsp. soy sauce
- ¼ tsp. garlic powder
- 1 tbsp. white vinegar
- 1 tbsp. brown sugar
- ½ fresh pineapple (peeled and cubed)
- 1 tbsp. tomato
- ¼ lb. fresh mushrooms, stems removed
- 1 green bell peppers, cut into 2 inch pieces
- ¼ cup lemon-lime flavored carbonated beverage
- ¼ tsp. pepper or to taste
- ¼ tsp. salt or to taste

DIRECTIONS

1. In a medium bowl, mix lemon-lime flavored carbonated beverage, brown sugar, soy sauce, garlic powder, white vinegar, salt and pepper.

2. Set aside about 1/2 cup of this marinade. Put steak in a large resealable plastic bag.

3. Cover with the remaining marinade, and seal. Refrigerate for 6/7 hours, or overnight.

4. Bring a saucepan of water to a boil. Add green peppers and cook for 45 seconds. Then drain and set aside.

5. Preheat grill for high heat. Thread tomatoes, steak, mushrooms, pineapple and green peppers onto skewers in an alternating. Discard marinade and the bag.

6. Lightly oil the grill grate. Cook kabobs on the prepared grill for 9-11 minutes, or to favorite doneness

7. cover frequently with reserved marinade during the last 4 minutes of cooking.

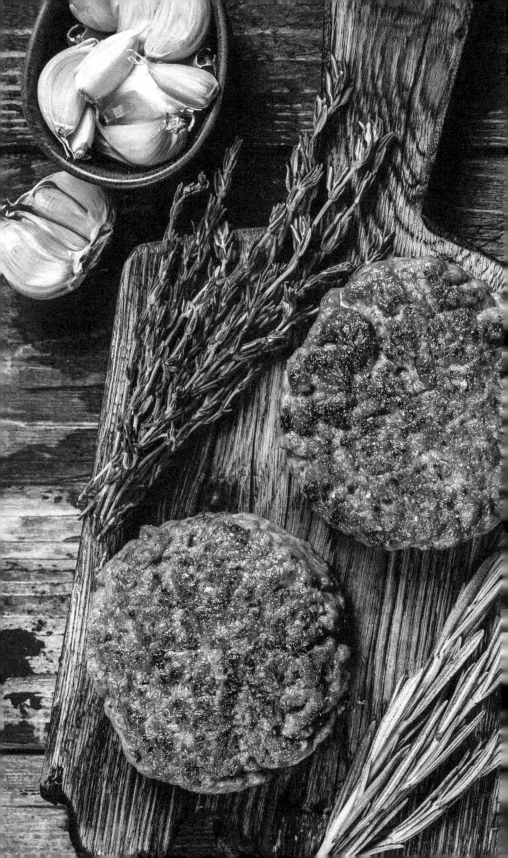

Burger Recipes

JUICY MOUTHWATERING BURGER

Prep. Time: 45 min   Cook Time: 10 min   Servings: 6

NUTRITION

Calories: 299 | Fat: 17g | Carbohydrates: 7g | Protein: 27g.

INGREDIENTS

- 2-pound ground beef
- 1 cup beer (your favorite one)
- 1 tsp. onion salt
- 1 tsp. garlic powder
- ¼ cup Worcestershire sauce
- Ground black pepper to taste

DIRECTIONS

1. Shape the ground beef into 3 patties. Put the patties in a dish.

2. Combine the Worcestershire sauce, garlic powder, onion salt, beer and pepper. Put the marinade over the burgers. Refrigerate for 20 minutes. Flip the burgers over and marinate for an additional 20 minutes.

3. Preheat an outdoor grill for medium-high heat, and lightly oil the grate

4. Place the patties on the hot grill and cook for a couple of minutes before flipping them over.

5. Cook the burgers to the favorite doneness, about 3/4 minutes per side for medium rare. The right temperature should be 150°F.

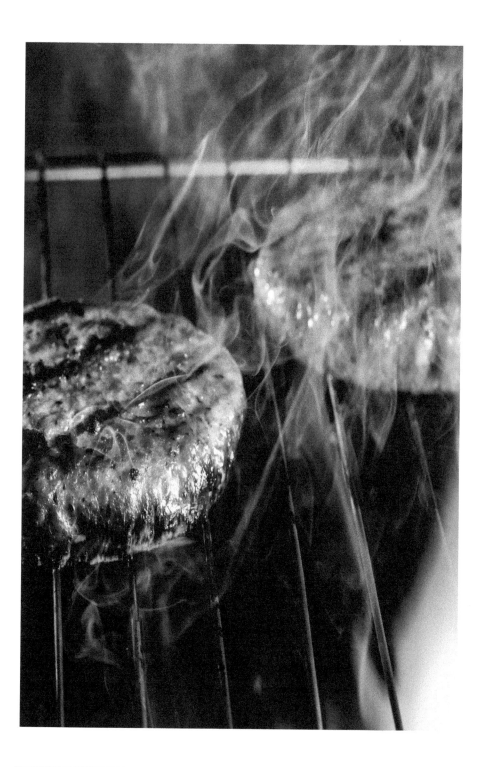

THE SPECIAL ONE

Prep. Time: 20 min   Cook Time: 10 min   Servings: 3

NUTRITION

Calories: 457 | Fat: 31g | Carbohydrates: 3g | Protein: 37g.

INGREDIENTS

- 1 lb. ground beef
- 1 egg
- 2 tbsp. Worcestershire sauce
- 2 tbsp. shredded Cheddar cheese
- ½ medium onion, chopped

DIRECTIONS

1. Preheat grill for high heat.

2. In a large bowl, combine together egg, the ground beef, Cheddar cheese, onion, and Worcestershire sauce using your hand. Create 3 large patties.

3. Place patties on the grill, and cook for 4 minutes per side, or until well done.

YOUR AMAZING HAMBURGER

Prep. Time: 15 min	Cook Time: 20 min	Servings: 8

NUTRITION

Calories: 437 | Fat: 23g | Carbohydrates: 9g | Protein: 41g.

INGREDIENTS

- 3 lb. lean ground beef
- Salt to taste
- Pepper to taste
- 1 tsp. dried rosemary
- 3 tsp. dried oregano
- 3 tsp. dried basil
- 1 onion, chopped
- 2 tsp. soy sauce
- 2 tsp. Worcestershire sauce
- 1 cup shredded cheddar cheese
- 2 tsp. dried parsley
- 2 tsp. garlic powder
- 2 clove garlic, minced
- 2 eggs

DIRECTIONS

1. Preheat a grill for high heat.

2. In a large bowl, combine together the onion, ground beef, soy sauce, cheese, eggs, Worcestershire sauce, garlic powder, garlic, oregano, parsley, basil, salt rosemary, and pepper.

3. Then form 4 patties.

4. Grill patties for 4 minutes per side on the hot grill, or until well cooked.

5. Serve on buns with your favorite adds.

QUICK AND EASY BURGER

Prep. Time: 20 min   Cook Time: 15 min   Servings: 6

NUTRITION

Calories: 297 | Fat: 19g | Carbohydrates: 9g | Protein: 29g.

INGREDIENTS

- 1½ lb. ground beef
- 1½ egg
- 1 tsp. salt
- 1 tsp. ground black pepper
- ¾ cup fine breadcrumbs

DIRECTIONS

1. Preheat an outdoor grill for high heat and lightly oil grate.

2. In a medium bowl, combine together salt, egg, and pepper. Put the ground beef and breadcrumbs into the mixture. Mix until blended with a fork. Form into 6 patties approximately 3 inches thick.

3. Place patties on the prepared grill. Cover and cook 6 to 8 minutes per side, or to desired doneness.

4. Place patties on the prepared grill. Cover and cook 7 to 9 minutes per side, or to favorite doneness.

5. You quick and easy burger is ready, enjoy!

BBE–BEST BURGER EVER

Prep. Time: 20 min   Cook Time: 10 min   Servings: 8

NUTRITION

Calories: 249 | Fat: 14g | Carbohydrates: 7g | Protein: 23g.

INGREDIENTS

- 2 lb. ground beef
- ¼ cup ketchup
- 2 eggs
- 2 tsp. ground black pepper
- ½ cup quick cooking oats
- 1 tsp. salt
- 2 tbsp. dried onion flakes.
- 2 tsp. dry onion soup mix

DIRECTIONS

1. Preheat an outdoor grill for high heat, and lightly oil grate.

2. In a large bowl, mix egg, quick cooking oats, ground beef, seasoning salt, dried onion flakes, ketchup, pepper, and dry onion soup mix.

3. Combine the mixture into about 8 burger patties.

4. Place burger patties on the prepared grill, and cook about 4 minutes on each side, to an internal temperature of 155° F. Enjoy!

THE BEST DOUBLE CHEESEBURGER

NUTRITION

Calories: 649 | Fat: 51g | Carbohydrates: 37g | Protein: 46g.

INGREDIENTS

- 1 lb. ground beef
- 3 hamburger buns, split
- 3 slice onion
- 3 slice tomato
- 3 leaf lettuce
- 3 tbsp. salad dressing
- 12 slices of melting cheese
- 2 tsp. salt

DIRECTIONS

1. Preheat a skillet over medium heat. Lightly toast both halves of the hamburger bun, cut sides down, a couple of minutes. Set aside.

2. Separate beef into 6 portions and form each into a thin patty slightly larger than the bun. Lightly salt each patty and cook on one side for a couple of minutes.

3. Flip patties over and immediately place two slices of American cheese on each one. Cook until meat has reached favorite doneness, a couple of minutes more. Temperature should reach 155°F.

4. Prepare the double cheeseburger in the following order: bottom bun, dressing, tomato, lettuce, beef patty with cheese, onion, beef patty with cheese, and top bun

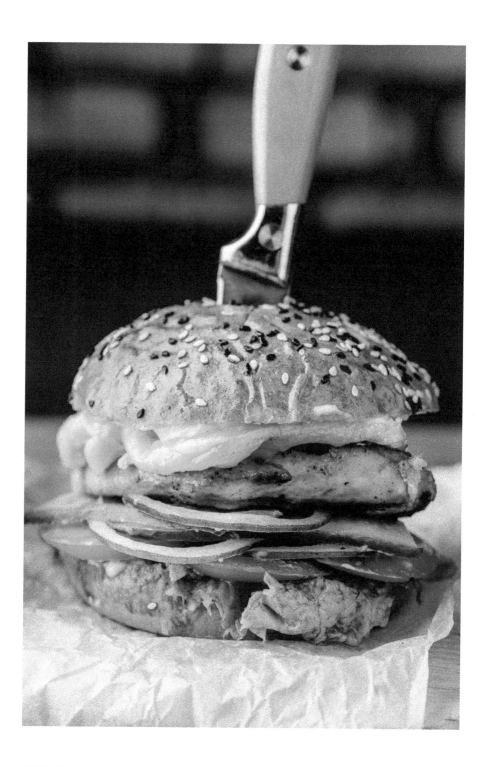

HEALTHY CHICKEN PARMESAN BURGER

Prep. Time: 14 min	Cook Time: 16 min	Servings: 8

INGREDIENTS

- 2-pound ground chicken
- 8 whole wheat hamburger buns, split
- 2 egg
- 2 cups chicken stock
- 1 cup seasoned breadcrumbs
- 8 slices provolone cheese
- 1 cup grated Parmesan cheese
- ⅓ cup spaghetti sauce, divided
- 2 cups crushed tomatoes
- 2 tbsp. Italian seasoning
- 2 onion, chopped
- 2 tsp. garlic powder
- 2 tbsp. olive oil
- 2 tsp. onion powder
- Salt, to taste
- Ground black pepper, to taste

DIRECTIONS

1. In a large bowl, combine egg, chicken, Parmesan cheese, breadcrumbs, Italian seasoning, 1 tablespoon spaghetti sauce, onion powder, and garlic powder. Season with pepper and salt.

2. Create mixture into 8 patties.

3. Press gently to flatten.

4. Heat 1 tablespoon olive oil in a large skillet.

5. Cook patties until browned, about 3 minutes per side. Transfer to a large plate.

6. Cook and mix onion in the drippings left in the skillet until translucent, about 4 minutes.

7. Add in remaining 2 tablespoons spaghetti sauce, chicken stock and crushed tomatoes. Cook until thickened and reduced by half, about 4 minutes.

8. Return patties to the skillet; cover with spaghetti sauce.

9. Place 1 slice of provolone cheese over each patty. Cover skillet and cook until cheese melts slightly, about a couple of minutes.

10. Place patties on buns; spoon tomato sauce on top

NUTRITION

Calories: 542 | Fat: 21g | Carbohydrates: 43g | Protein: 45g.

EXOTIC CILANTRO CHICKEN BURGERS

Prep. Time: 20 min	Cook Time: 10 min	Servings:8

NUTRITION

Calories: 426 | Fat: 19g | Carbohydrates: 29g | Protein: 33g.

INGREDIENTS

- 2-pound ground chicken
- ½ cup ranch dressing, or to taste
- 1 cup chopped fresh cilantro
- 2 avocado, peeled, and sliced
- 2 tbsp. soy sauce
- Hamburger buns
- 2 tbsp. garlic powder
- Cooking spray
- 2 tsp. lime juice
- 2 tbsp. ground black pepper
- 2 tsp. ground ginger

DIRECTIONS

1. In a large bowl, mix together ground chicken, soy sauce, garlic powder, cilantro, lime juice, ground black pepper and ground ginger.

2. Form the mixture into 8 patties.

3. Prepare a skillet with cooking spray and place over medium heat.

4. Cook burgers in the hot skillet until cooked through and no longer pink in the middle, about 4 minutes per side. Perfect temperature should be 165° F.

5. Serve on hamburger buns with slices of avocado and a 1 tablespoon ranch dressing

SPICY CHICKEN BURGERS

Prep. Time: 30 min   Cook Time: 10 min   Servings: 8

NUTRITION

Calories: 783 | Fat: 31g | Carbohydrates: 88g | Protein: 49g.

INGREDIENTS

- 2 large tomato, sliced
- 2 tbsp. chili powder
- 8 whole wheat rolls
- 1 tbsp. ground cumin
- 1 tbsp. minced garlic
- ⅓ cup shredded cabbage
- 2-pound ground chicken.
- 2 eggs
- 8-oz. light sour cream
- 2 tsp. ground black pepper
- 2 large avocado - halved, and peeled
- ½ tsp. garlic powder
- 1½ tbsp. salt

DIRECTIONS

1. In a small bowl, combine together chili powder, cumin, 1½ teaspoon salt, black pepper and minced garlic.

2. In a large bowl, sprinkle 3/4 of the chili powder mixture over ground chicken. Add egg; mix well and shape into 8 patties.

3. Preheat grill for medium heat and lightly oil the grate. Grill patties until browned and juices run clear, about 4 minutes per side. The right temperature should be 160°F.

4. In a small bowl, mash avocado and season with garlic powder and ½ teaspoon salt.

5. In a bowl, combine sour cream, remaining chili powder mixture, and shredded cabbage together to make coleslaw.

6. Toast rolls lightly on the grill. Place chicken patties on the buns. Top each patty with mashed avocado, sliced tomato and a large scoop of coleslaw.

BACON CHEDDAR BURGERS

NUTRITION

Calories: 437 | Fat: 24g | Carbohydrates: 21g | Protein: 33g.

INGREDIENTS

- 2-lbs. ground beef
- 8 hamburger buns
- 1 cup shredded Cheddar cheese
- 1 cup real bacon bits
- ¼ cup prepared horseradish
- 1 tsp. garlic powder
- 1 tsp. pepper
- 1 tsp. salt

DIRECTIONS

1. Preheat grill for high heat.

2. In a large bowl, combine together Cheddar cheese, the ground beef, salt, horseradish, pepper, bacon bits and garlic powder, using your hands. Shape the mixture into 8 hamburger patties.

3. Lightly oil the grill grate. Place hamburger patties on the grill, and cook for 4 minutes per side, or until well done. Serve on buns

VEGGIE MUSHROOM HAMBURGER

Prep. Time: 15 min   Cook Time: 15 min   Servings: 3

NUTRITION

Calories: 249 | Fat: 13g | Carbohydrates: 21g | Protein: 13g.

INGREDIENTS

- 1½ packages sliced mushrooms
- 4 tbsp. olive oil
- ¼ cup shredded Parmigiano-Reggiano cheese
- ¼ onion, finely chopped
- 1 egg
- 2 cloves garlic, minced
- ⅓ cup dry breadcrumbs
- ½ tsp. salt
- ¼ cup rolled oats
- ¼ tsp. black pepper
- ¼ tsp. dried oregano

DIRECTIONS

1. Heat olive oil in a large skillet over medium heat

2. Then add onion, garlic, and mushrooms to the hot oil and season with oregano, salt, and black pepper.

3. Cook and mix mushroom mixture until mushrooms have given up their juice and the juice has almost evaporated, about 8-9 minutes.

4. Then, put cooked mushrooms to a cutting board and chop into small pieces with a knife.

5. Transfer mushrooms to a large bowl. Combine in rolled oats and breadcrumbs.

6. Stir Parmigiano-Reggiano cheese into the mixture, followed by egg.

7. Let mixture stand for about 20 minutes.

8. Moisten hands with a little bit of water, pick up about 1/4 cup of mixture, and form into burgers.

9. Heat remaining 2 tablespoons olive oil in a skillet over medium heat.

10. Pan-fry burgers until browned and cooked through, 4 to 5 minutes.

VEGETARIAN BBB: BLACK BEAN BURGER

Prep. Time: 25 min	Cook Time: 49 min	Servings: 3

NUTRITION

Calories: 218 | Fat: 2g | Carbohydrates: 47g | Protein: 13g.

INGREDIENTS

- 15-oz. black beans, rinsed and drained
- ½ large, sweet potato
- ½ cooking spray
- 1 tsp. ground cinnamon
- 1 tsp. salt
- 1 tsp. freshly grated ginger
- ½ tsp. ground cumin
- 1 tsp. mustard
- 2 tsp. chopped onion
- ¼ cup quick cooking oats

DIRECTIONS

1. Preheat oven to 400° F.

2. Poke holes into sweet potato with a fork; and place on a greased baking sheet.

3. Bake in the preheated oven until sweet potato can be easily pierced with a fork, about 40 minutes.

4. Remove from oven and cool until easily handled.

5. Reduce heat to 340° F.

6. Spray a baking sheet with cooking spray

7. Into a large bowl, put the peel sweet potato.

8. Add black beans and mash with a fork.

9. Add onions, oats, cumin, mustard, salt, ginger, and cinnamon and combine until well mixed.

10. Shape mixture into 3 patties with wet hands and place onto prepared baking sheet.

11. Bake in the preheated oven until cooked in the center and crisp on the outside, about 7 minutes on each side.

QUICK FALAFEL BURGER

Prep. Times: 20 min   Cook Times: 15 min   Servings: 6

NUTRITION

Calories 234 | Fat: 12g | Carbs:29g | Protein: 9g.

INGREDIENTS

- 3 tbsp. olive oil, divided
- ⅓ cup dry breadcrumbs
- 1½ small red onion, chopped
- 1 tsp. salt
- 1½ large garlic clove, minced
- 1 tbsp. lemon juice
- 1½ large garlic clove, minced
- 1½ can spinach, well drained
- 1½ can garbanzo beans, drained and rinsed
- 6 hamburger buns
- Tzatziki sauce to taste
- Lettuce leaves
- 8 tomatoes, sliced
- Red onion, sliced

DIRECTIONS

1. In a skillet over medium heat, in 1 tablespoon hot olive oil, cook garlic and red onion about 4 minutes or until tender-crisp.

2. To food processor, add 1/4 of garbanzo beans, salt, and lemon juice; pulse canned spinach until mixture is a smooth paste.

3. Add remaining breadcrumbs, onion mixture and garbanzo beans; pulse until coarsely chopped.

4. Shape mixture into 6 patties. (If desired, you can refrigerate until ready to cook.) In a skillet over medium heat, in remaining tablespoon hot olive oil, cook falafel patties until golden and crisp, turning once.

5. Add tomatoes, lettuce leaves, onions and Tzatziki sauce to taste. Enjoy!

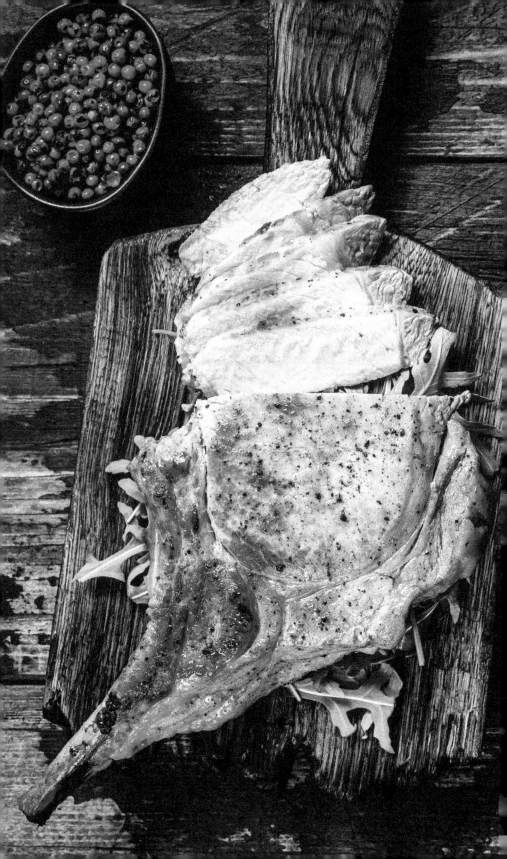

Pork Recipes

AMAZING PORK FOR BURRITOS & TACOS

Prep. Time: 30 min   Cook Time: 8 hours   Servings: 6

NUTRITION

Calories: 347 | Fat: 13g | Carbs: 31g | Protein: 24g.

INGREDIENTS

- 1½ pounds pork shoulder roast
- 7-oz. chopped green chilies
- 2 tbsp. salsa
- 1 tbsp. taco seasoning mix.
- 1 bottle cola
- 2 tbsp. brown sugar
- 1.30-oz. packet fajita seasoning

DIRECTIONS

1. Place pork roast in the crock of a slow cooker and add 4 cups water. Cook on High for about 5 hours.

2. Remove pork from the slow cooker and drain liquid. Cut the pork into 4 pieces and set aside.

3. Puree salsa in the blender.

4. Combine cola, the pureed salsa, fajita seasoning, brown sugar, green chilies and taco seasoning, in the crock of the slow cooker.

5. Add the pork and cook on High for about 3 hours more.

6. Remove the pork and serve. Enjoy!

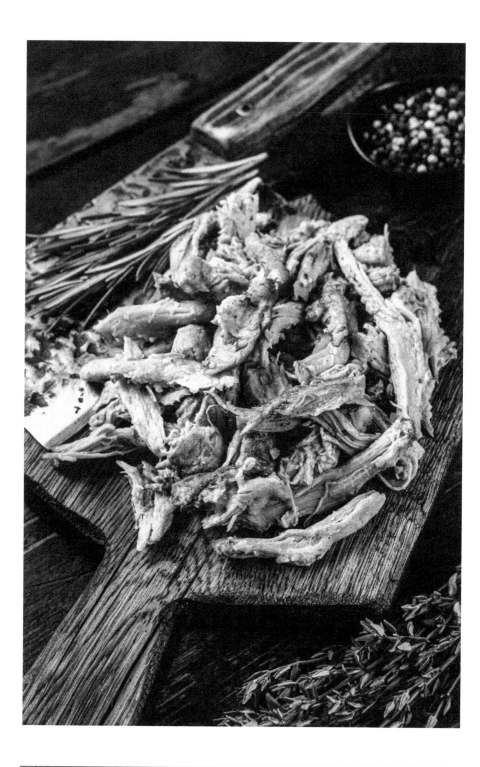

IRONMAN PULLED PORK

Prep. Time: 25 min	Cook Time: 10 hours	Servings: 9

NUTRITION

Calories: 367 | Protein: 24g | Carbs: 22g | Fat: 24g.

INGREDIENTS

- 2½ lb. pork shoulder roast
- ½ cup water
- 2 tsp. steak seasoning
- 1 bottle barbeque sauce
- 1½ pounds boneless pork ribs
- ½ tsp. Worcestershire sauce
- ¼ tsp. smoked paprika
- ½ tsp. dried chipotle chili pepper
- 1 tsp. soy sauce

DIRECTIONS

1. Season pork roast with half the steak seasoning and place in the center of a slow cooker.

2. Layer about 1/2 the pork rib meat around pork roast and season with about half the remaining chili pepper, paprika and steak seasoning.

3. Layer the remaining pork ribs in the slower and season with the remaining steak seasoning.

4. Add Worcestershire sauce and soy sauce.

5. Slowly pour water over pork.

6. Cook on Low for about 10 hours.

7. Then, put the meat to a roasting pan; remove and discard every bones and large chunks of fat. Shred pork with forks.

8. Drain and discard liquid from slow cooker; wipe away any remaining fat.

9. Return shredded pork to slow cooker and add about 1/2 bottles barbeque sauce. Then mix.

10. Continue to heat on Low until ready to serve. Serve with the other 1/2 bottle barbeque sauce.

EASY SUPER(B) PULLED PORK

Prep. Times: 15 min	Cook Times: 3 h 40 min	Servings: 6

NUTRITION

Calories: 658 | Fat: 43g | Carbs: 27g | Protein: 43g.

INGREDIENTS

- 3 lb. Boston butt roast
- ½ onion, chopped
- 3 tbsp. barbecue sauce
- 2 cloves garlic, minced
- ¼ tsp. cayenne pepper
- 1 tsp. ground black pepper
- 1 tsp. salt

DIRECTIONS

1. Rub garlic, pepper and seasoning salt, and cayenne pepper to taste onto roast.

2. Place roast in a large oven and fill half way with water; add onion. Bring to a rolling boil over high heat. Reduce heat simmer and let cook until meat falls off the bone. This should take about 3 hours and half / 4 hours.

3. Place hot roast in a serving bowl and pour on your favorite barbecue sauce. Mix until blended. Serve on your favorite buns.

BBQ PORK FOR SANDWICHES (SLOW COOKING)

| 15 min | 7 hours | 6 |

NUTRITION

Calories: 221 | Fat: 9g | Carbs: 23g | Protein: 13g.

INGREDIENTS

- 1-pound boneless pork roast
- 1 bottle BBQ sauce (your favorite one)
- Ground black pepper to taste
- Salt to taste
- 1 tsp. crushed red pepper flakes
- 2 tbsp. black coffee
- ½ small onion, diced
- 1 tbsp. Worcestershire sauce
- ½ cup water
- 1 tbsp. bourbon whiskey
- 3 tbsp. beef broth
- 5 cloves garlic

DIRECTIONS

1. Season the roast with black pepper and salt. Put the seasoned roast, Worcestershire sauce, coffee, garlic, bourbon whiskey, onion, beef broth, water, and red pepper flakes in a slow cooker set to LOW.

2. Cook about 4 hours. Scoop garlic cloves out of the cooker and mash with a fork; then return the mashed garlic to the slow cooker. Cook another 3 to 3 hours and a half.

3. Place the roast to a large cutting board, and discard liquid. Shred the roast into strands using 2 forks and return meat to the slow cooker.

4. Add the barbeque sauce and continue cooking on LOW for 1 hour and a half to 3 hours.

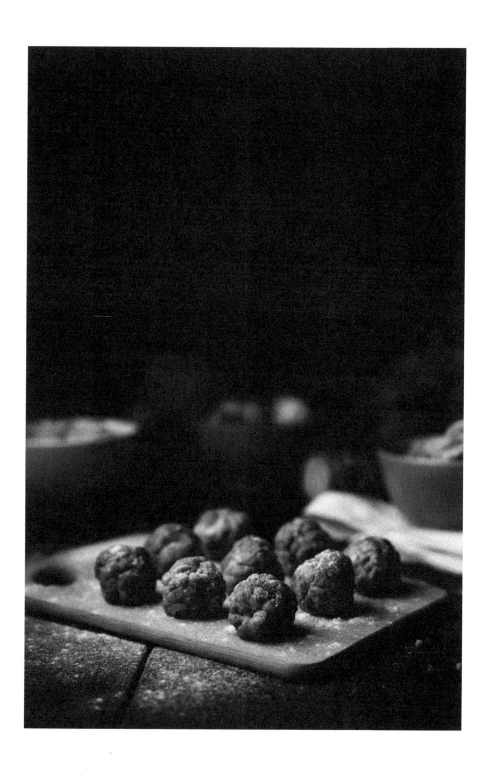

TASTY SAUSAGE BALLS

Prep. Time: 15 min   Cook Time: 20 min   Servings: 24 sausage balls

NUTRITION

Calories: 180 | Fat: 8g | Carbs: 3g | Protein: 24g.

INGREDIENTS

- 0.8 lb. ground pork sausage
- 3 tbsp. biscuit baking mix
- 0.8 lb. Cheddar cheese, shredded

DIRECTIONS

1. Preheat oven to 355 degrees F

2. In a large bowl, combine cheese, biscuit baking mix and sausage. Form into walnut size balls and place on baking sheets.

3. Bake in preheated oven for about 25 minutes, until golden brown and sausage is cooked.

GRILLED PORK TENDERLOINS

| Prep. Times: 10 min | Cook Times: 25 min | Servings: 4 |

NUTRITION

Calories 194 | Fat: 5g | Carbs: 16g | Protein: 25g.

INGREDIENTS

- 3 tbsp. honey
- Hot cooked rice
- 3 tbsp. low-sodium soy sauce
- 1 (1 lb.) pork tenderloin
- 3 tbsp. teriyaki sauce
- ⅛ tsp. black ground pepper
- 1 tbsp. brown sugar
- ¼ tsp. ground cinnamon
- ½ tbsp. minced fresh gingerroot
- ¼ tsp. onion powder
- 2 tsp. ketchup
- 1½ garlic cloves, minced

DIRECTIONS

1. In a large bowl, combine honey, soy sauce, teriyaki sauce, brown sugar, ginger root, garlic cloves, ketchup, onion powder cinnamon and pepper.

2. Pour half of the marinade into a bowl; add tenderloins and turn to coat.

3. Cover and refrigerate 7/8 hours or overnight, turning pork occasionally.

4. Cover and refrigerate remaining marinade.

5. Drain pork, discarding marinade.

6. Grill, covered, over indirect medium-hot heat for 25-30 minutes or until a thermometer reads 145°F, turning occasionally and basting with reserved marinade.

7. Let stand 4-5 minutes before slicing. Serve with rice.

GRILLED PORK CHOPS

Prep. Times: 120 min	Cook Times: 10 min	Servings: 12

NUTRITION

Calories 367 | Fat: 23g | Carbs:3g | Protein: 39g.

INGREDIENTS

- 1 cups water
- 12 boneless pork loin chops, trimmed of fat
- ⅔ cup light soy sauce
- 1 tbsp. minced garlic
- ½ cup vegetable oil
- ⅓ cup lemon pepper seasoning

DIRECTIONS

1. In a deep bowl, stir soy sauce, water, vegetable oil, minced garlic, and lemon pepper seasoning; add pork chops and marinate in refrigerator at least a couple of hours.

2. Preheat an outdoor grill for medium-high heat and lightly oil the grate.

3. Remove pork chops from the marinade and shake off excess. Then discard the remaining marinade.

4. Cook the pork chops on the preheated grill until no longer pink in the center, about 6 minutes per side (an instant-read thermometer inserted into the center should read 150°F).

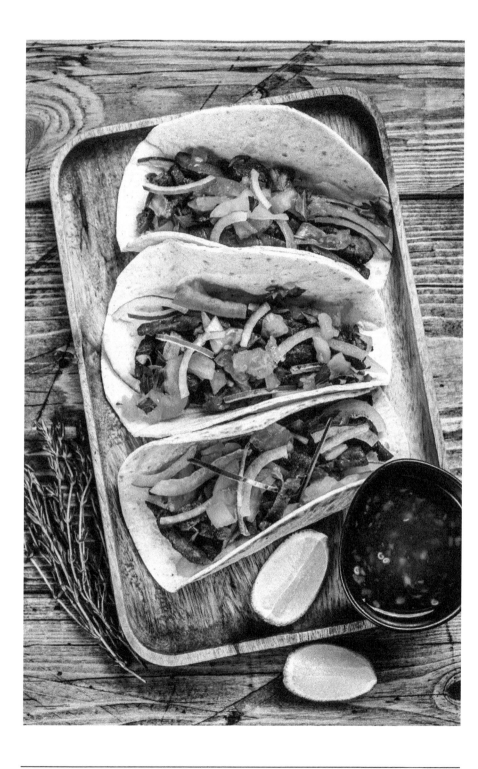

MEXICAN PORK TACOS

Prep. Time: 25 min	Cook Time: 40 min	Servings: 9

INGREDIENTS

- 15 spicy chiles
- 3 tbsp vegetable oil
- 1½ skinless pork butt, cut into 1/2-inch cubes
- 1½ chipotle pepper
- Adobo with Pepper, to taste
- 1½ medium white onion, halved
- 1 tsp. cumin
- 1½ Pineapple Chunks
- 3 tbsp. Minced Garlic
- ⅓ cup white vinegar

To Garnish:

- 10-ounce Corn Tortillas, warmed
- 3 tbsp. finely chopped fresh cilantro
- ½ lime, cut into wedges

DIRECTIONS

1. Bring 2 cups water to boil in medium saucepan over medium-high heat. Add chiles. Reduce heat to medium-low and simmer until chiles soften, about 9/10 minutes; transfer to plate.

2. Remove and discard stem and seeds. Meanwhile, coarsely chop one onion half; reserve remaining half. Strain pineapples; reserve juice and fruit separately.

3. Transfer chiles, chopped onion half, vinegar, reserved pineapple juice, cumin and garlic to bowl of food processor. Puree until smooth, about a couple of minutes. Transfer chile mixture to saucepan over medium-high heat. Bring chile mixture to a boil; cook until paste loses raw onion taste, about a couple of minutes.

4. Season with Adobo; cool. In large container with lid, or in large ziptop bag, combine pork cubes, cooled chile marinade and reserved pineapple chunks; transfer to refrigerator. Marinate at least a couple of hours, or up to 20 hours.

5. Heat oil in large skillet over medium-high heat. Strain pork and pineapples, discarding marinade. Add pineapples and pork to skillet.

6. Cook in batches until dark golden brown on all sides and cooked through, about 13-15 minutes; then transfer to large serving plate.

7. Meanwhile, finely slice remaining onion half. Then, Transfer sliced onion to bowl with cilantro. Serve pineapple mixture and pork and in warm tortillas. Garnish pork tacos with onions, cilantro, and limes.

NUTRITION

Calories: 297 | Fat: 14g | Carbs: 3g | Protein: 27g.

SUMMER BBQ TERIYAKY PORK KABOBS

Prep. Times: 30 min	Cook Times: 20 min	Servings: 8

INGREDIENTS

- ¼ cup soy sauce
- 16 bite-size chunks fresh pineapple
- ¼ cup olive oil
- 16 cherry tomatoes
- 1½ large red onion, cut into 12 wedges
- 1 tsp. crushed red pepper flakes
- 4 portobello mushrooms, cut into quarters
- ½ tsp. ground ginger
- 3 garlic cloves, minced
- Salt, to taste
- Pepper, to taste
- 1⅓ lb. boneless pork loin, cut into 1-inch cubes
- 1 tbsp. brown sugar
- 14 oz. low-sodium beef broth
- 2 tbsp. cornstarch
- 2 tbsp. soy sauce

DIRECTIONS

1. In a shallow dish, stir together olive oil, 3 tablespoons soy sauce, red pepper flakes, 1 clove minced garlic, salt, and pepper. Add pork cubes and turn to coat evenly with marinade.

2. Cover, and refrigerate for about 4 hours.

3. In a saucepan, mix cornstarch, beef broth, 2 cloves minced garlic, brown sugar, 2 tablespoons soy sauce, and ginger. Bring to a boil, stirring constantly. Reduce heat, and simmer about 5 minutes.

4. Preheat an outdoor grill for high heat and lightly oil grate. Thread pork cubes onto skewers, alternating with mushrooms, tomatoes, onion, and pineapple chunks.

5. Cook on grill for 14/15 minutes, or until meat is cooked through. Turn skewers and baste often with sauce during cooking.

NUTRITION

Calories 293 | Fat: 16g | Carbs:19g | Protein: 21g.

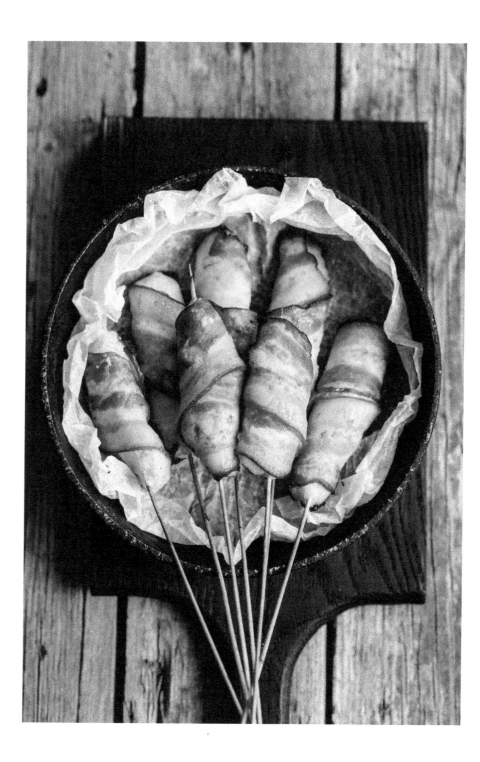

EASY BACON JALAPENO WRAPS

Prep. Times: 10 min   Cook Times: 10 MIN   Servings: 8

NUTRITION

Calories 389 | Fat: 37g | Carbs:3g | Protein: 11g.

INGREDIENTS

- 8 fresh jalapeno peppers, halved lengthwise and seeded
- 16 slices bacon
- 8 oz. cream cheese

DIRECTIONS

1. Preheat an outdoor grill for high heat.

2. Spread cream cheese to fill 1/2 jalapeno. Wrap with bacon. Then secure with a toothpick.

3. Place on the grill and cook about 10 minutes or until bacon is crispy.

ASIAN PORK CHOPS

Prep. Times: 20 min   Cook Times: 15 min   Servings: 12

NUTRITION

Calories 179 | Fat: 7g | Carbs:12g | Protein: 20g.

INGREDIENTS

- 1 cup soy sauce
- 12 boneless pork chops
- ½ cup brown sugar
- ¼ tsp. garlic powder
- 1 tsp. ground ginger
- 2 tbsp. vegetable oil
- ¼ cup lemon juice

DIRECTIONS

1. In a bowl, stir the soy sauce, lemon juice, brown sugar, ginger, garlic powder and vegetable oil. Set aside some of the mixture in a separate bowl for marinating during cooking.

2. Pierce the pork chops on both sides with a fork, place in a large resealable plastic bag, and cover with the remaining marinade mixture. Refrigerate about 7 hours.

3. Preheat the grill for high heat.

4. Lightly oil the grill grate. Discard marinade, and grill pork chops about 7 minutes per side, or to your favorite doneness, marinating often with the reserved portion of the marinade.

FINGERLICKING BOURBON RIBS

| Prep. Times: 15 min | Cook Times: 1 hour | Servings: 9 |

NUTRITION

Calories 643 | Fat: 27g | Carbs:39g | Protein: 45g.

INGREDIENTS

- 1½ cup dark brown sugar
- 4½ lb. country style pork ribs
- 1 cup bourbon
- 6 garlic cloves
- 1½ cup light soy sauce

DIRECTIONS

1. Process bourbon, brown sugar, garlic and soy sauce, in a blender to mince garlic with other ingredients.

2. Pour over ribs and marinate for plenty of hours in the refrigerator.

3. Preheat an outdoor grill for medium heat, and lightly oil grate.

4. Put ribs on grate, and cover. Cook 50 minutes to 1 hour depending on thickness of your ribs.

5. When finished, the internal temperature of the ribs should be 165° F

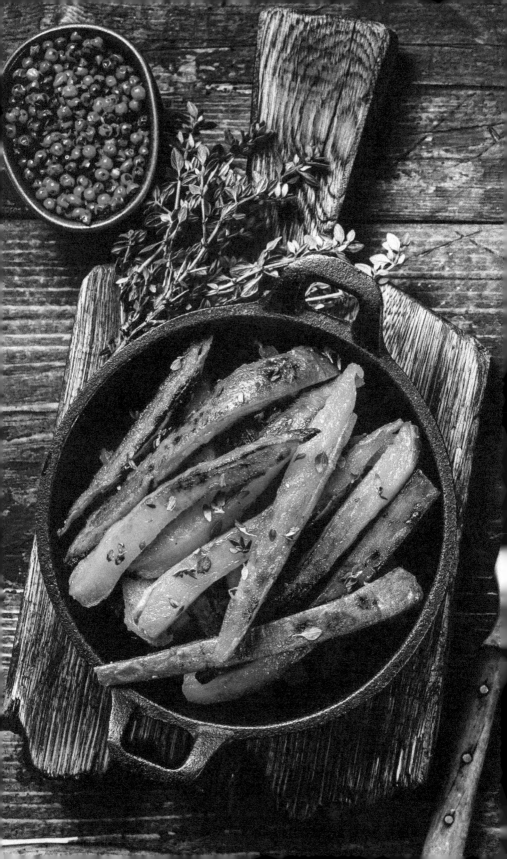

Veggies Recipes

TASTY GRILLED SALAD

Prep. Time: 18 min	Cook Time: 10 min	Servings: 3

NUTRITION

Calories: 233 | Fats: 18g | Carbs: 14g | Protein: 4g.

INGREDIENTS

- ½ lb. fresh asparagus, trimmed
- Salt, to taste
- Black pepper, to taste
- 1 zucchini
- 1 yellow squash
- 1 tsp. prepared mustard
- ¼ cup extra-virgin olive oil
- 2 tbsp. red wine vinegar
- ½ large red onion, sliced
- 1 red bell pepper

DIRECTIONS

1. Preheat grill for medium heat and lightly oil the grate

2. Place zucchini, asparagus, red onion, yellow squash, and red bell peppers on preheated grill; cook until vegetables are tender and slightly charred, for about 12 to 15 minutes. Then, remove vegetables from grill and cut into bite-sized pieces.

3. Stir together in a bowl red wine vinegar, mustard, olive oil, salt, pepper and garlic to make the dressing. Mix vegetables with dressing in a bowl.

4. Serve at room temperature or warm if desired.

GRILLED VEGETARIAN SANDWICH

Prep. Time: 15 min	Cook Time: 5-7 min	Servings: 4

NUTRITION

Calories: 698 | Fats: 28g | Carbs: 77g | Protein: 34g.

INGREDIENTS

- 1 zucchini, cut
- 4 tomatoes, sliced
- 1 small eggplant
- 8 oz. fresh mozzarella, sliced
- 2 red bell pepper, quartered
- ½ cup basil pesto
- 2 small whole-grain baguette
- 1 tbsp. olive oil
- Pepper to taste
- 1 tsp. salt

DIRECTIONS

1. Mix red bell pepper, zucchini, and eggplant, in a bowl. Sprinkle salt over the mixture. Set aside to allow the vegetables to tenderize, about 4 hours.

2. Preheat grill for medium heat and lightly oil the grate.

3. Drain moisture from vegetable mixture. Brush vegetables with olive oil to coat; season with black pepper.

4. Cook vegetables on hot grill until tender, a couple of minutes per side. Then, transfer to a bowl and set aside.

5. Toast cut sides of baguette 1 to 2 minutes. Spread basil pesto evenly over toasted surface, then arrange grilled vegetables.

6. Top each with sliced mozzarella and plum tomato slices; top sandwich with the remaining baguette pieces. Enjoy!

ITALIAN VEGETABLES SANDWICH

Prep. Time: 20 min   Cook Time: 35 min   Servings: 8

NUTRITION

Calories: Calories: 348 | Fats: 15g | Carbs: 47g | Protein: 10g.

INGREDIENTS

- 1½ eggplant, sliced
- 1 lb. loaf focaccia bread
- 3 red bell peppers
- ¼ cup mayonnaise
- 2 tbsp. olive oil
- 4 garlic cloves, crushed
- 3 portobello mushrooms, sliced

DIRECTIONS

1. Preheat oven to 380°F

2. Brush red bell peppers and eggplant with 1 to 2 tablespoon olive oil. Put on a baking sheet and roast in preheated oven. Roast eggplant until tender, about 20 to 25 minutes; roast peppers until blackened. Remove from oven and set aside to cool.

3. Heat 1 tablespoon olive oil and cook and stir mushrooms until tender. Mix crushed garlic into mayonnaise. Slice focaccia and spread mayonnaise mixture on both halves.

4. Peel cooled peppers, and slice. Place peppers, eggplant, and mushrooms on focaccia and serve.

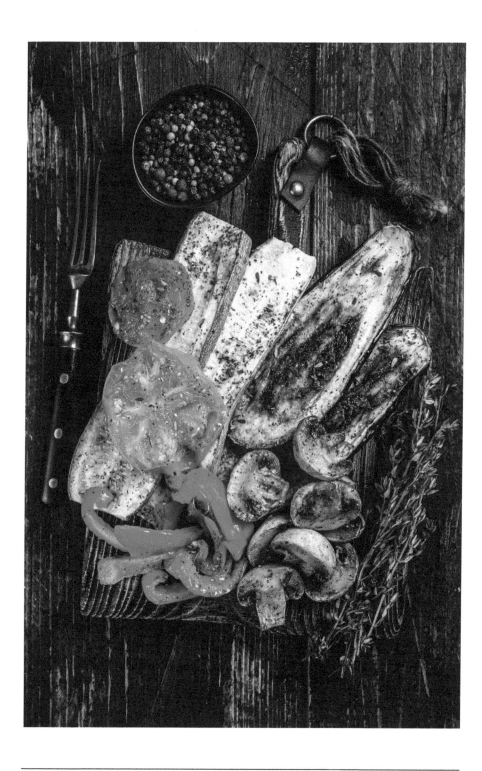

EASY QUICK GRILLED VEGETABLES

Prep. Time: 15 min	Cook Time: 10 min	Servings: 9

INGREDIENTS

- 3 yellow squash, sliced
- 1½ medium yellow bell pepper, chopped
- 3 zucchini, sliced
- 1½ medium red bell pepper, chopped
- 1½ medium orange bell pepper, chopped
- 1½ medium green bell pepper, chopped
- 1 tbsp. balsamic vinegar
- 1 tsp. sea salt
- 1 tsp. black pepper
- 1 cup sliced sweet onion
- 2 cups sliced portobello mushrooms
- ¼ cup olive oil
- 3 tbsp. garlic and herb seasoning blend
- 2 tsp. olive oil

DIRECTIONS

1. Preheat an outdoor grill for high heat.

2. Mix zucchini, yellow squash, onion, bell peppers, and mushrooms in a large bowl. Toss with 2/3 tablespoons olive oil, balsamic vinegar, garlic, salt, and pepper.

3. Heat 1 teaspoon olive oil in a grill-safe pan on the preheated grill. Add veggies and grill, mixing continuously, until zucchini, squash and peppers are still slightly crunchy, 9 to 11 minutes.

NUTRITION

Calories: 116 | Fat: 7g |Carbs: 12g | Protein: 3g.

GRILLED VEGETABLE SKEWERS

Prep. Time: 10 min   Cook Time: 10 min   Servings: 6

NUTRITION

Calories: 403 | Fats: 18g | Carbs: 59g | Protein: 8g.

INGREDIENTS

- 12 wooden skewers
- ⅓ tsp. ground black pepper
- 3 zucchini
- 2 tsp. dried oregano
- 3 yellow squash, cut
- ½ cup olive oil
- 2 tsp. dried basil
- ¾ lb. whole fresh mushrooms
- 1½ red bell pepper, cut into chunks
- 1½ fresh pineapple, cut
- 18 cherry tomatoes
- 1½ red onion, cut
- 1 tsp- salt

DIRECTIONS

1. Soak skewers in water for about 15 minutes

2. Preheat grill for medium heat and lightly oil the grate. Alternately thread yellow squash slices, zucchini slices, onion, mushrooms, tomatoes, pineapple, and bell pepper onto the skewers.

3. Mix in a bowl olive basil, oil, salt, black pepper and oregano; brush mixture over vegetables.

4. Cook skewers on preheated grill until vegetables are tender, turning and basting vegetables with olive oil mixture occasionally, 12 to 14 minutes.

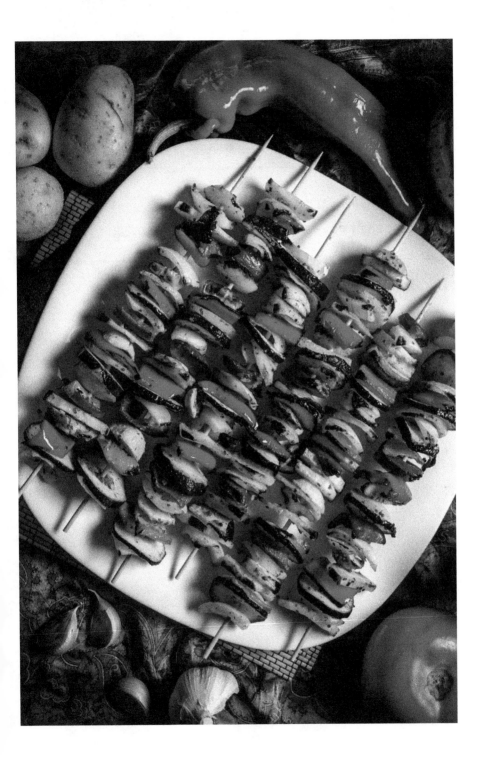

EASY GRILLED ONION & POTATOES

Prep. Time: 10 min   Cook Time: 30 min   Servings: 6

NUTRITION

Calories: 281 | Fats: 12g | Carbs: 39g | Protein: 5g.

INGREDIENTS

- ⅓ cup butter
- 6 medium potatoes, sliced
- 2 tsp. ground black pepper
- 2 tsp. salt
- 2 red onions, sliced

DIRECTIONS

1. Preheat grill for medium heat.

2. Wrap the vegetables into 2 or 3 squares of aluminum foil and lay one on top of the other.

3. Place some onion and potatoes in the middle, sprinkle with pepper and salt, and dot with butter.

4. Wrap and seal the edges.

5. Repeat with remaining potatoes and onion.

6. Place aluminum wrapped package over indirect heat, and cover. Cook for half an hour, turning once.

7. Serve warm. Enjoy!

EASY CHEESY POTATOES

| Prep. Time: 15 min | Cook Time: 30 min | Servings: 4 |

NUTRITION

Calories: 293 | Fat: 15g | Carbs: 32g | Protein: 7g.

INGREDIENTS

- 4 potatoes, sliced
- Salt, to taste
- Grand black pepper, to taste
- 2 tbsp. diced onion
- 1 tbsp. cold butter
- ½ cup shredded Cheddar cheese
- ½ cup shredded Mozzarella cheese
- 2 tbsp. grated Parmesan cheese

DIRECTIONS

1. Cut 2 lengths of heavy-duty foil, placing one on top of the other. Spray top one with non-stick spray. Spread potatoes on foil leaving plenty of room to fold up later.

2. Put butter and onions over potatoes; then layer the Mozzarella, Cheddar cheese and Parmesan, over the potatoes; season with salt and pepper. Bring opposite edges of foil together and seal.

3. Place the packet directly onto your fire and cook until the potatoes are soft, about 30- 35 minutes.

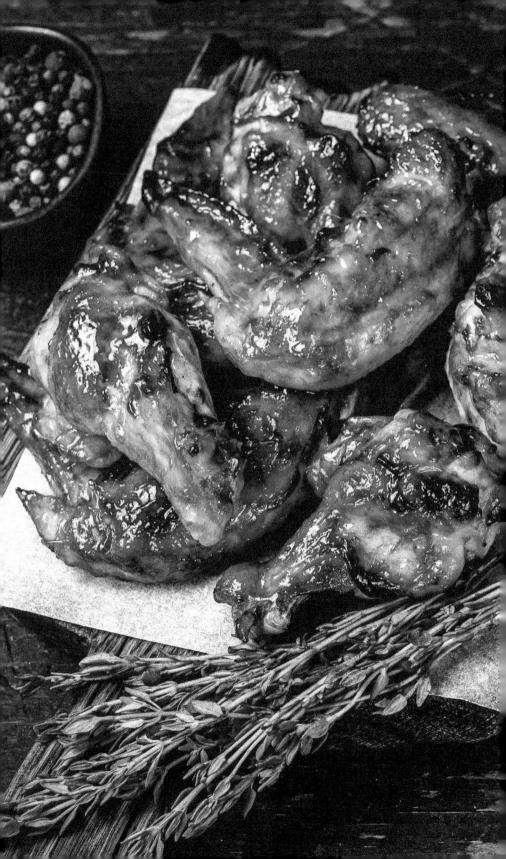

Chicken Recipes

TASTY CHICKEN TERIYAKI

Prep. Time: 20 min   Cook Time: 15 min   Servings: 8

NUTRITION

Calories: 238 | Fat: 8g | Carbohydrates: 17g | Protein: 24g.

INGREDIENTS

- 8 skinless, boneless chicken breast halves
- 1 tbsp. sesame oil
- 2 cups teriyaki sauce
- 1 tbsp. minced fresh garlic
- ½ cup lemon juice

DIRECTIONS

1. Put teriyaki sauce, chicken, garlic, lemon juice, and sesame oil in a large resealable plastic bag. Seal bag and shake to coat.

2. Place in refrigerator for 1 day, turning occasionally.

3. Preheat grill for high heat.

4. Lightly oil the grill grate.

5. Remove chicken from bag, discarding any remaining marinade.

6. Grill for about 7 minutes each side, or until juices run clear when chicken is pierced with a fork.

EASY CHICKEN TACO

Prep. Time: 25 min   Cook Time: 20 min   Servings: 8

INGREDIENTS

- 15-oz. black beans, rinsed and drained
- 1 tbsp. olive oil
- 1 cup medium-hot salsa
- ½ tsp. cayenne pepper
- ½ cup chopped fresh cilantro
- ⅓ cup sour cream
- 1½ lime, cut into wedges
- 1 tbsp. lime juice
- 3 tbsp. chili powder
- 1½ lime, cut into wedges
- 1½ avocado - peeled, pitted, and sliced
- ¾ cup shredded lettuce
- 6 corn tortillas
- 1½ pound skinless, boneless chicken breast halves
- 1 tsp. brown sugar
- 1 tsp. ground coriander
- 1 tsp. ground cumin

DIRECTIONS

1. Preheat an outdoor grill for medium-high heat and lightly oil the grate.

2. Stir salsa, black beans, 1/2 cup cilantro, and lime juice in a bowl; set aside.

3. Mix chili powder, cayenne pepper, coriander, cumin, brown sugar, and olive oil in a bowl until smooth; rub mixture over chicken breasts.

4. Cook chicken breasts on preheated grill until no longer pink in the center and the juices run clear, about 11 minutes per side (at least 165° F). While the chicken is cooking, place tortillas on grill and grill until lightly brown on both sides, about 4 minutes.

5. Put chicken to a cutting board and slice into long thin strips. Divide chicken strips over tortillas and top with lettuce, bean mixture, and remaining half cup cilantro. Serve with lime wedges, sour cream, and avocado.

NUTRITION

Calories: 464 | Fat: 19g | Carbohydrates: 43g | Protein: 36g.

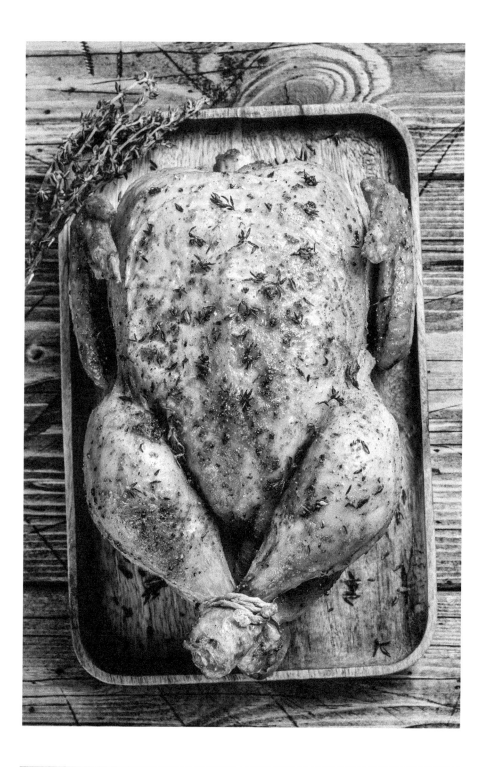

YOGURT SMOKY CHICKEN

Prep. Time: 20 min	Cook Time: 35 min	Servings: 4

NUTRITION

Calories: 511 | Fat: 28g | Carbohydrates: 6g | Protein: 54g.

INGREDIENTS

- ¼ cup low-fat Greek yogurt
- 2 tsp. salt
- ⅓ lemon, juiced
- 1 tsp. harissa
- 2 tsp. lemon zest
- 2 tsp. lemon juice
- 2 tsp. olive oil
- 5-lb. whole chicken, cut into 4 pieces
- 1 tsp. ground black pepper
- 1 tsp. herbs de Provence
- 2 tsp. paprika
- 3 garlic cloves, crushed

DIRECTIONS

1. Mix together the 1/8 cup yogurt, paprika, a teaspoon of salt, the juice from 1/2 lemon, lemon zest, garlic, olive oil, herbs de Provence, and black pepper in a bowl.

2. Pour into a resealable plastic bag. Add chicken, coat with the marinade, squeeze out excess air, and seal the bag.

3. Marinate in refrigerator for about 4 hours.

4. Preheat an outdoor grill for medium-high heat, and lightly oil the grate.

5. Combine 1 tablespoon lemon juice, 1/8 cup yogurt, and harissa in a small bowl. Set aside.

6. Remove chicken from bag and transfer to a plate or baking sheet lined with paper towels. Pat chicken pieces dry with more paper towels. Season with 1 tsp salt.

7. Grill chicken, skin-side down, on the preheated grill for a couple of minutes. Turn each piece and move to indirect heat.

8. Grill, turning often, with lid down until well-browned and meat is no longer pink in the center, about 30 minutes. (ideal temperature should be 160°F)

9. Serve chicken with the yogurt harissa mixture on the side. Enjoy!

EASY DUMPLINGS & BACON CHICKEN

Prep. Time: 25 min	Cook Time: 30 min	Servings: 6

NUTRITION

Calories: 448 | Fat: 21g | Carbs: 45g | Protein: 24g.

INGREDIENTS

- 2 slices bacon
- ¾ cup milk
- 2 large potatoes, peeled and diced
- 2 tbsp. biscuit mix
- ¾ onion, diced
- 3 skinless, boneless chicken breast halves - diced
- ¾ can whole kernel corn, drained and rinsed
- ¼ cup chicken broth
- Pepper, to taste
- Salt, to taste
- ¾ tsp. poultry seasoning
- ¼ cup half-and-half

DIRECTIONS

1. Put bacon in a deep skillet. Cook over medium high heat until evenly brown. Drain, crumble and set aside; then reserve bacon drippings in skillet.

2. Add chicken, onion and potatoes, to bacon drippings and cook for about 15 minutes, mixing occasionally. Pour in chicken broth; season with pepper, salt and poultry seasoning. Then add corn, and simmer all together for about 15 minutes.

3. Pour in half-and-half and bring to a boil; add crumbled bacon. In a medium bowl, combine milk with biscuit mix and mix very well (dough should be thick).

4. Drop tablespoon sizes of dough into boiling mixture; reduce heat and simmer for about 10 minutes uncovered, then another about 10 minutes covered. (Note for you: Do not mix while simmering, or dumplings will break apart).

5. Serve hot. Enjoy!

SPARTAN GRILLED CHICKEN

| Prep. Time: 20 min | Cook Time: 20 min | Servings: 4 |

NUTRITION

Calories: 441 | Fat: 28g | Carbohydrates: 6g | Protein: 39g.

INGREDIENTS

- 4 garlic cloves, minced
- ⅔ lemon, cut into wedges
- 1 tbsp. dried oregano
- 4 chicken leg quarters
- 1 tsp. red pepper flakes
- 2 tsp. white vinegar
- 1 tsp. ground black pepper
- ¼ cup lemon juice
- 2 tbsp. olive oil

DIRECTIONS

1. In a large bowl mix together vinegar, lemon juice, garlic, red pepper flakes, olive oil, oregano, black pepper, and vinegar

2. Make 2 slashes on the skin side down to the bone in the thigh section and 1 in the leg section of each leg quarter. Season both sides of chicken generously with salt.

3. Transfer to bowl with marinade coat all sides. Cover and marinate in refrigerator 5 to 10 hours.

4. Transfer chicken to paper-towel-lined sheet pan to drain slightly.

5. Place leg quarters on grill skin side down over semi-direct heat and cook about 7 minutes.

6. Turn chicken and cook another 7 minutes.

7. Continue cooking and turning until internal temperature reaches 160°F, about 7-9 minutes more. Serve with lemon wedges. Enjoy!

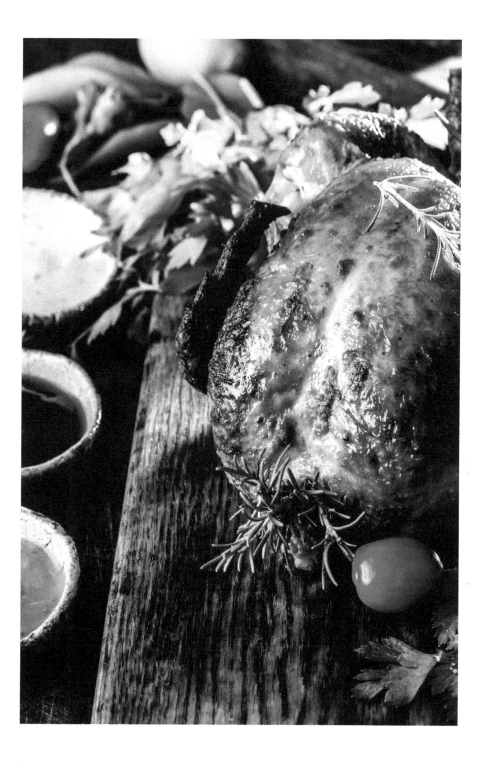

CHINESE SPICY GRILLED CHICKEN

Prep. Time: 20 min	Cook Time: 50 min	Servings: 12

NUTRITION

Calories: 478 | Fat: 26g | Carbs: 5g | Protein: 52g.

INGREDIENTS

- 2 (5-lb.) whole chickens, cut in half
- 2 tsp. hot chile paste
- 1 lime, juiced
- 2 tsp. fish sauce
- 6 garlic cloves, crushed
- 2 tsp. Chinese five-spice powder
- ⅔ cup seasoned rice vinegar
- 2 tsp. soy sauce
- 2 tbsp. seasoned rice vinegar
- 1 tbsp. hot chile paste
- 2 tbsp. fish sauce

DIRECTIONS

1. Score the skin side of each piece of chicken a couple of times

2. Mix together 1 tablespoon fish sauce, ginger, soy sauce, the juice of 1/2 lime, 1 tablespoon rice vinegar, garlic, Chinese five-spice powder, and 2 teaspoons hot chile paste in a bowl. Pour into a resealable plastic bag.

3. Add chicken, coat evenly with the marinade, squeeze out excess air, and seal the bag.

4. Marinate in refrigerator for about 6 hours.

5. Preheat an outdoor grill for medium-high heat, and lightly oil the grate.

6. Remove chicken halves from the bag and transfer to a plate lined with paper towels. Pat chicken pieces dry with more paper towels. Then, reserve marinade mixture in a small bowl.

7. Mix together juice of 1/2 lime, the 1/3 cup rice vinegar, 1 teaspoon hot chile paste, and 1 teaspoon fish sauce in a small bowl. Set aside.

8. Grill chicken, skin-side down, on the preheated grill for a couple of minutes. Turn each piece, brush with reserved marinade mixture, and move to indirect heat.

9. Grill, brushing with glaze and turning ever 11-14 minutes, until well-browned and meat is no longer pink in the center, about 40-45 minutes total (ideal temperature should be 180°F).

10. Pour vinegar lime juice mixture over the chicken and serve. Enjoy!

BEST GRILLED CHICKEN EVER

| Prep. Time: 15 min | Cook Time: 35 min | Servings: 6 |

NUTRITION

Calories: 321 | Fat: 23g | Carbohydrates: 4g | Protein: 22g.

INGREDIENTS

- 2 tbsp. white vinegar
- 2 chicken leg quarters
- 2 tbsp. water
- 1 (8-oz.) bone-in chicken breasts
- 1 sticks butter
- 1 tsp. minced garlic
- 2 tbsp. Worcestershire sauce
- 2 tsp. white sugar
- 2 tbsp. garlic salt
- 1 tbsp. ground black pepper

DIRECTIONS

1. Mix water, vinegar, Worcestershire sauce, butter, sugar, garlic salt, pepper, and minced garlic in a pot. Bring to a boil. Remove from heat and let marinade cool to room temperature, at least 40 minutes.

2. Place chicken in a resealable zip-top bag. Pour marinade over chicken, seal, and marinate, 9 hours to overnight.

3. Preheat an outdoor grill for medium-high heat and lightly oil the grate.

4. Put chicken pieces to the grill, shaking off excess marinade; then discard remaining marinade.

5. Grill chicken until no longer pink in the center, 35 to 45 minutes (ideal temperature should be at least 160°F).

MARINATED CHICKEN KABOOBS

Prep. Time: 25 min	Cook Time: 15 min	Servings: 8

NUTRITION

Calories: 241 | Fat: 8g | Carbohydrates: 13g | Protein: 32g.

INGREDIENTS

- 8 oz. fat-free plain yogurt
- 2 large green bell pepper, cut into 1½-inch pieces
- ⅔ cup crumbled feta cheese with basil and sun-dried tomatoes
- 2 large red onion, cut into wedges
- 1 tsp. lemon zest
- 2 lb. skinless, boneless chicken breast - cut into 1-inch pieces
- ½ tsp. crushed dried rosemary
- ½ tsp. ground black pepper
- 1 tsp. salt
- 1 tbsp. dried oregano
- ¼ cup fresh lemon juice

DIRECTIONS

1. In a large baking dish, mix feta cheese, yogurt, lemon zest, lemon juice, salt, pepper, oregano, and rosemary. Place the chicken in the dish and turn to coat. Cover, and marinate about 4 hours in the refrigerator.

2. Preheat an outdoor grill for high heat.

3. Thread the chicken, green bell pepper pieces and onion wedges alternately onto skewers. Discard remaining yogurt mixture.

4. Grill skewers on the prepared grill until the chicken is no longer pink and juices run clear. Enjoy!

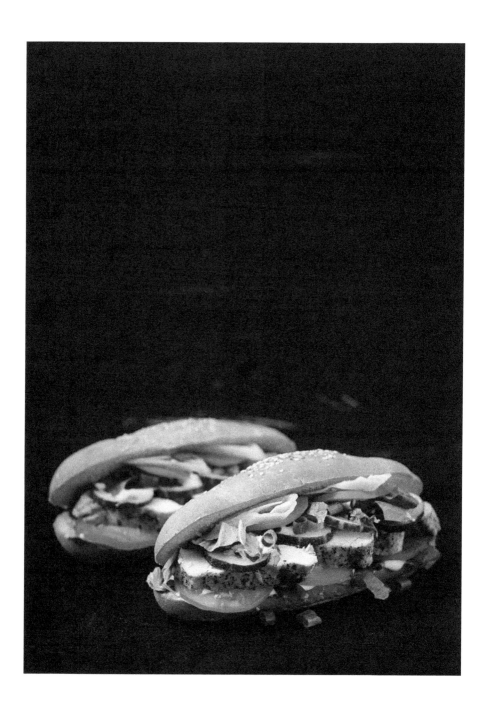

YUMMY CHICKEN BREAST SANDWICH

Prep. Time: 20 min   Cook Time: 15 min   Servings: 6

NUTRITION

Calories: 638 | Fat: 33g | Carbohydrates: 49g | Protein: 36g.

INGREDIENTS

- 6 skinless, boneless chicken breast halves
- 6 your favorite sandwich bread, split
- 12 thin slices Monterey Jack cheese
- 1½ cup chipotle BBQ sauce
- 1 tsp. salt
- 1½ avocado, sliced
- 1 tbsp. spicy seasoning
- ¾ lime, juiced
- 1½ jalapeno pepper, seeded and sliced
- ⅓ cup olive oil

DIRECTIONS

1. Slice a small pocket into each chicken breast. Layer avocado slices, sliced jalapeno and cheese slices, inside the chicken pockets.

2. Pinch chicken breasts closed and secure with skewers or toothpicks; put chicken into a bowl.

3. Combine together in a bowl spicy seasoning, lime juice, olive oil, and salt; drizzle half of the mixture over chicken breasts. Turn chicken breasts over and drizzle with remaining olive oil mixture.

4. Cover and refrigerate for about half an hour.

5. Preheat an outdoor grill for high heat, and lightly oil the grate.

6. Place chicken breasts on preheated grill and cook for 6-7 minutes; turn chicken over and brush with BBQ sauce on the cooked side.

7. Continue grilling for about 4-5 minutes; turn chicken over and apply BBQ sauce to the second cooked side.

8. Cook chicken until no longer pink in the center and the juices run clear, about a couple of minutes more (ideal temperature should be at least 160°F).

9. Make the sandwich and serve. Enjoy!

FINGERLICKING CHICKEN BREAST

| Prep. Time: 20 min | Cook Time: 10 min | Servings: 6 |

NUTRITION

Calories: 240 | Fat: 14g | Carbohydrates: 2g | Protein: 25g.

INGREDIENTS

- 1½ lb. skinless, boneless chicken breast halves, cut into cubes
- Ground black pepper to taste
- ½ cup fresh onion juice
- ¼ cup butter, melted
- 2 tbsp. olive oil
- 1 tsp. salt
- 2 tbsp. olive oil
- 1 tsp. curry

DIRECTIONS

1. Mix, in a large bowl lime juice, olive oil, fresh onion juice, salt and pepper.

2. Mix in the cubes of chicken. Cover, and store in the refrigerator overnight.

3. The day after, put the cubes of chicken onto skewers for grilling. Brush each side with melted butter.

4. Cook on the grill over medium heat until the chicken turns golden brown.

SMOKY HERBY CHICHEN

Prep. Time: 20 min   Cook Time: 4 hours   Servings: 4

NUTRITION

Calories: 319 | Fat: 22g | Carbohydrates: 2g | Protein: 31g.

INGREDIENTS

- ½ (4-lb.) whole chicken
- 2 tsp. fresh chives, finely chopped
- 1 tbsp. butter
- 1 tsp. chopped fresh basil
- 1 tsp. chopped fresh oregano
- 1 tsp. chopped fresh parsley

DIRECTIONS

1. Preheat an outdoor grill for low heat.

2. Rinse chicken inside and out. Pat dry. Loosen skin around the breast area.

3. Combine herbs together and place half under the skin and the other half inside the chicken. Put butter in various places under the skin.

4. Cook chicken with smoke for about 4 hours or until juices run clear when poked with a fork. Enjoy!

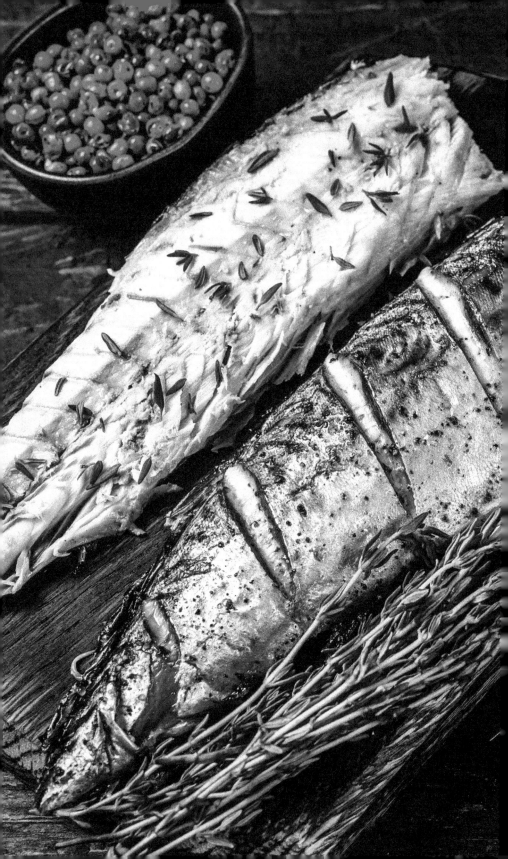

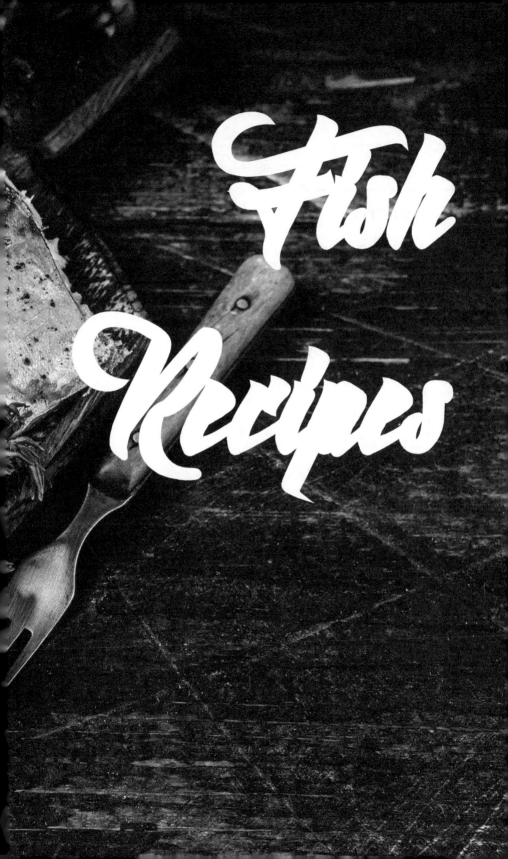

SESAME GRILLED SALMON STAKE

Prep. Times: 15 min   Cook Times: 10 min   Servings: 4

NUTRITION

Calories: 398 | Fat: 19g | Carbs: 15g | Protein: 44g.

INGREDIENTS

- ½ cup light soy sauce
- 1 tbsp. sesame seeds
- 3 tbsp. honey
- 2 tsp. sesame oil
- 2 lb. salmon fillets
- 2 garlic cloves, minced
- 2 tbsp. grated fresh ginger

DIRECTIONS

1. In a bowl mix together ginger, honey, soy sauce, and garlic until marinade is evenly mixed. Set aside 1/3 of the marinade.

2. Place salmon fillets in shallow dish; pour the remaining marinade over the salmon. Cover dish with plastic wrap and refrigerate for about 6 minutes.

3. Heat sesame oil in a large skillet over medium-high heat.

4. Remove salmon from marinade, shaking to remove excess marinade, and put it, skin-side up, into the hot oil; cook for about 4 minutes.

5. Discard unused marinade in the shallow dish. Flip salmon and drizzle the reserved 1/3 of the marinade over salmon; sprinkle with sesame seeds.

6. Cook until fish flakes easily with a fork, about 6 minutes. Flip salmon, remove skin, and cook one minute more.

MEDITERRANEAN GRILLED SALMON WITH AVOCADO DIP

Prep. Time: 20 min	Cook Time: 15 min	Servings: 3

NUTRITION

Calories: 392 | Fat: 27g | Carbs: 7g | Protein: 33g.

INGREDIENTS

- 1 avocado - peeled, pitted and diced
- 1 tsp. salt
- Pepper to taste
- 1 tsp. lemon pepper
- 1 tsp. dried dill weed
- 1 garlic clove, peeled and minced
- 1 tbsp. Greek-style yogurt
- 1 lb. salmon steaks
- 1 tsp. fresh lemon juice

DIRECTIONS

1. Preheat an outdoor grill for high heat, and lightly oil grate.

2. Mash together garlic, yogurt, avocados, and lemon juice, in a bowl. Season with pepper and salt.

3. Rub salmon with lemon pepper, salt, and dill. Place on the prepared grill, and cook about 15 minutes, turning once, until easily flaked with a fork.

4. Serve with the avocado mixture.

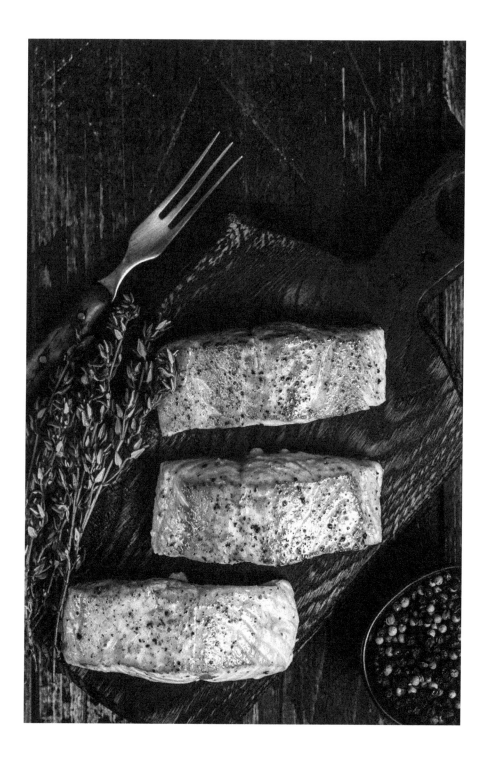

QUICK TASTY GRILLED SALMON

Prep. Time: 15 min	Cook Time: 20 hours	Servings: 4

NUTRITION

Calories: 268 | Protein: 31g | Carbs: 17g | Fat: 10g.

INGREDIENTS

- ⅓ cup soy sauce
- 4 (5-oz.) salmon fillets
- ¼ cup pure maple syrup
- 1 tsp. salt
- 1 tsp. ground black pepper
- 2 garlic cloves, minced
- 1 tbsp. minced fresh ginger root

DIRECTIONS

1. Stir soy maple syrup, sauce, ginger, garlic, pepper, and salt in a shallow container with a tight-fitting lid.

2. Put salmon, flesh-side down, in the container and seal.

3. Marinate in the refrigerator for about 35 minutes.

4. Preheat an outdoor grill for high heat and lightly oil the grate. Once heated, turn down one side to low heat.

5. Place salmon, skin-side down, over low heat on the preheated grill and close the lid.

6. Allow to cook, basting once with reserved marinade, until easily flaked with a fork, 18 to 22 minutes. Then remove from the grill by sliding a spatula between salmon and the skin.

SUMMER GRILLED TUNA STEAKS

NUTRITION

Calories: 351 | Fat: 7g | Carbs: 19g | Protein: 55g.

INGREDIENTS

- ⅓ cup red seedless grapes, halved
- ⅓ cup fresh lemon juice
- ½ cup capers, drained and rinsed
- 6 (8-oz) tuna steaks
- 1½ shallot, minced
- Salt, to taste
- Black pepper, to taste
- 3 tbsp. chopped fresh parsley
- 1 tbsp. olive oil

DIRECTIONS

1. Preheat an outdoor grill for medium-high heat and lightly oil grate.

2. Mix together in a bowl capers, grapes, parsley, shallot, and olive oil; season to taste with salt and pepper and set aside.

3. Place tuna steaks onto a plate, and brush with lemon juice. Season with salt and pepper to taste.

4. Cook tuna steaks on preheated grill until cooked to desired degree of doneness, a couple of minutes per side for medium-rare.

5. Serve with caper salsa and grape.

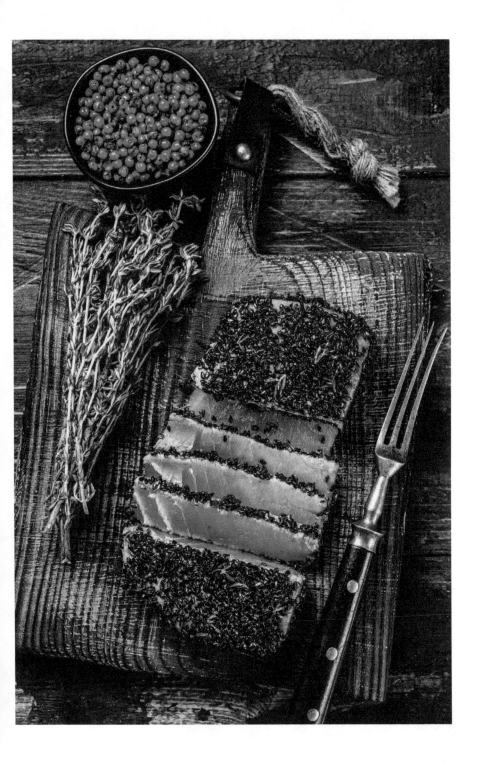

SALMON STEAK WITH BLUEBERRY SAUCE

Prep. Times: 15 min	Cook Times: 15 min	Servings: 6

NUTRITION

Calories 377 | Fat: 24g | Carbs:13g | Protein: 28g.

INGREDIENTS

- ¾ cup chicken stock
- Salt, to taste
- Pepper, to taste
- ⅓ cup balsamic vinegar
- 3 tbsp. olive oil
- ⅓ cup orange juice
- 6 (6-oz) salmon steaks
- 1 tsp. honey
- 1 tbsp. cornstarch
- 1 tbsp. chopped fresh chives
- ⅓ cup chicken stock
- 1½ cup fresh blueberries

DIRECTIONS

1. Pour vinegar, orange juice, 1/2 cup chicken stock, and honey into a saucepan. Bring to a boil over high heat, then reduce heat to medium. Dissolve cornstarch in 1/4 cup of chicken stock and mix into the simmering sauce.

2. Cook and mix until the sauce turns clear, about a couple of minutes. Stir in chives and the blueberries and keep warm over low heat.

3. Preheat grill to medium high heat.

4. Brush salmon with oil, and season to taste with salt and pepper. Grill until the fish flakes easily with a fork, about 4 minutes per side.

5. Serve with blueberry sauce. Enjoy!

GRILLED FISH TACOS WITH DRESSING

| Prep. Time: 40 min | Cook Time: 10 min | Servings:12 |

NUTRITION

Calories: 407 | Fat: 21g | Carbs: 37g | Protein: 32g.

INGREDIENTS

- ½ cup extra virgin olive oil
- 2 lb. tilapia fillets, cut into chunks
- ¼ cup distilled vinegar
- 2 tsp. hot pepper sauce
- ¼ cup fresh lime juice
- 1 tsp. ground black pepper
- 1 tbsp. lime zest
- 2 tsp. seafood seasoning
- 1 tsp. chili powder
- 1 tbsp. honey
- 4 garlic cloves, minced
- 1 tsp. cumin

Dressing:

- 8 oz. light sour cream
- Salt, to taste
- Black pepper, to taste
- 1 cups adobo sauce from chipotle peppers
- 1 tsp. seafood seasoning
- ¼ cup fresh lime juice
- ½ tsp. chili powder
- ½ tsp. cumin
- 1 tbsp. lime zest

Toppings:

- 2 package tortillas
- 4 limes, cut in wedges
- 6 ripe tomatoes, seeded and diced
- 2 small head cabbage, shredded
- 2 bunches cilantro, chopped

DIRECTIONS

For Marinade:

1. Mix in a bowl together the vinegar, cumin, olive oil, lime juice, honey, lime zest, hot sauce, garlic, seafood seasoning, chili powder, and black pepper, until blended.

2. Place the tilapia in a shallow dish and pour the marinade over the fish.

3. Cover, and refrigerate 7 to 8 hours.

For Dressing:

4. In a bowl combine the sour cream and adobo sauce. Mix in the lime zest, chili powder, lime juice, cumin, seafood seasoning. Add salt, and pepper (to taste).

5. Cover, and refrigerate until needed.

6. Preheat an outdoor grill for high heat and lightly oil grate. Set grate 4 inches from the heat.

7. Remove fish from marinade, drain off any excess and discard marinade.

8. Grill fish pieces until easily flaked with a fork, turning once, about 8-10 minutes.

9. Assemble tacos by placing fish pieces in the center of tortillas with desired amounts of cilantro, cabbage, and tomatoes; drizzle with dressing.

10. To serve, roll up tortillas around fillings, and garnish with lime wedges.

SUMMER GRILLED HALIBUT

Prep. Times: 25 min   Cook Times: 10 min   Servings: 6

NUTRITION

Calories 273 | Fat: 14g | Carbs: 4g | Protein: 36.

INGREDIENTS

- 6 (6-oz.) fillets halibut
- 1 tbsp. olive oil
- 1½ lime, cut into wedges
- 3 tbsp. butter
- Salt to taste
- Pepper to taste
- 1 tbsp. fresh lime juice
- 4 garlic cloves, coarsely chopped
- ¾ cup chopped fresh cilantro

DIRECTIONS

1. Preheat a grill for high heat.

2. Squeeze the juice from the lime wedges over fish fillets, then season them with pepper and salt.

3. Grill fish fillets for about 4/5 minutes on each side, until browned and fish can be flaked with a fork.

4. Heat the oil in a skillet over medium heat. Add the garlic; cook and mix until fragrant, about a couple of minutes. Combine in the butter, remaining cilantro and lime juice.

5. Serve halibut with the cilantro butter sauce.

FLAVORFUL GRILLED TROUT

Prep. Time: 20 min	Cook Time: 15 min	Servings: 8

NUTRITION

Calories: 239 | Fat: 12g | Carbs: 4g | Protein: 29g.

INGREDIENTS

- 4 whole trout, cleaned
- 4 sprigs fresh thyme
- 2 tbsp. olive oil, divided
- 4 sprigs fresh rosemary
- 2 pinch salt or to taste
- 2 pinch ground black pepper
- 2 garlic cloves, minced
- 1 sweet onion, thinly sliced
- 1 lemon, thinly sliced

DIRECTIONS

1. Preheat an outdoor grill for high heat and lightly oil the grate.

2. Rub each trout generously with olive oil and sprinkle with salt; sprinkle inside of cavities with salt and black pepper. Place onion slices and 1/2 lemon into cavity of each trout, along with minced garlic, and place a sprig of rosemary and thyme into cavities.

3. Turn preheated grill down to low and place the trout directly onto the grill; cook until the skins are browned, about 7 minutes per side, flipping once.

PARTY SALMON SKEWERS

Prep. Times: 15 min   Cook Times: 10 min   Servings: 6

NUTRITION

Calories 91 | Fat: 4g | Carbs:9g | Protein: 8g.

INGREDIENTS

- ½ lb. salmon filet without skin
- 6 skewers
- 6 fresh lemon wedges
- 2 tbsp. soy sauce
- 1 tsp. ground black pepper
- ½ fresh garlic clove, minced
- 2 tbsp. honey
- 1 tsp. vinegar
- ½ tsp. minced fresh ginger root

DIRECTIONS

1. Slice salmon lengthwise into 6 long strips, and thread each onto a soaked wooden skewer.

2. Mix together in a bowl, honey, soy sauce, vinegar, garlic, ginger, and pepper. pour over skewers, turning to coat. Let stand at room temperature for about 40 minutes.

3. When finished marinating, transfer marinade to a small saucepan, and simmer for about 5 minutes.

4. Preheat an outdoor grill for medium-high heat.

5. Lightly oil grill grate. thread 1 lemon wedge onto the end of each skewer.

6. Cook skewers on the preheated grill for about 4 minutes per side, brushing often with marinade, or until fish flakes easily with a fork.

GRILLED BLACKENED FISH SANDWICHES

Prep. Times: 15 min	Cook Times: 10 min	Servings: 4

INGREDIENTS

- ½ (14-oz.) package coleslaw mix
- Salt, to taste
- Ground black pepper, to taste
- ¼ small red onion, chopped
- ⅛ tsp. celery seed
- 2 tbsp. apple cider vinegar
- ¼ tsp. white sugar
- 1 tbsp. Creole mustard
- 2 tbsp. olive oil

Fish:

- 1 lb. cod fillets
- 4 hamburger buns
- 1 tbsp. blackening seasoning
- 1 tsp. olive oil
- 1 tsp. paprika

DIRECTIONS

1. Combine in a large bowl coleslaw mix, celery seed, vinegar, onion, oil, sugar, mustard, salt, and pepper. Mix until evenly combined. Set aside.

2. Place cod fillets on a clean work surface. Sprinkle 1/2 of the paprika and 1/2 of the blackening seasoning over the fillets.

3. Flip fillets over and sprinkle with remaining blackening seasoning and paprika. Brush olive oil over both sides of the fillets.

4. Preheat an outdoor grill for medium-high heat and lightly oil the grate.

5. Grill fish for about 3 minutes. Flip and grill for about 3 minutes more.

6. Cut fillets in 1/2 and place each half on a hamburger bun. Top with slaw. Enjoy!

NUTRITION

Calories 338 | Fat: 13g | Carbs:30g | Protein: 24g.

GRILLED COD
IN ASIAN MARINADE

Prep. Times: 15 min   Cook Times: 10 min   Servings: 4

NUTRITION

Calories 271 | Fat: 2g | Carbs: 31g | Protein: 34g.

INGREDIENTS

- 1 cup olive oil
- 6 (4-oz.) tilapia fillets
- ¾ cup finely chopped fresh parsley
- 1½ pinch sea salt to taste
- ⅓ cup balsamic vinegar
- 2 tsp. hot pepper sauce
- 1 tsp. ground black pepper
- ¾ lemon, juiced
- 3 garlic cloves, minced
- 1 tbsp. dried oregano

DIRECTIONS

1. Place cod in a gallon-sized freezer bag. Add green onions, lemon juice, orange juice, brown sugar, soy sauce, ginger paste, and garlic; stir to combine.

2. Squeeze excess air out of the bag and seal. Marinate in the refrigerator for at least a couple of hours.

3. Preheat an outdoor grill for medium-high heat and lightly oil the grate.

4. Place cod in a grill basket and cook on the preheated grill until internal temperature of fish reaches 135°F, about 8 minutes.

TASTY GRILLED TILAPIA

Prep. Times: 15 min	Cook Times: 10 min	Servings: 6

NUTRITION

Calories 476 | Fat: 41g | Carbs: 5g | Protein: 24g.

INGREDIENTS

- 1 cup olive oil
- 6 (4-oz.) tilapia fillets
- ¾ cup finely chopped fresh parsley
- 1½ pinch sea salt to taste
- ⅓ cup balsamic vinegar
- 2 tsp. hot pepper sauce
- 1 tsp. ground black pepper
- ¾ lemon, juiced
- 3 garlic cloves, minced
- 1 tbsp. dried oregano

DIRECTIONS

1. Mix olive oil, parsley, garlic, vinegar, lemon juice, black pepper, oregano, hot sauce, and sea salt in a large, zip-top bag. Shake well. Add tilapia fillets and marinate in the mixture for 35/40 minutes.

2. Preheat an outdoor grill for high heat and lightly oil the grate.

3. Cook fillets on the preheated grill until they flake easily with a fork, about 4/5 minutes per side.

BEST GRILLED MARINATED SHRIMP EVER

Prep. Time: 35 min	Cook Time: 10 min	Servings: 12

NUTRITION

Calories: 439 | Fat: 38g | Carbohydrates: 4g | Protein: 26g.

INGREDIENTS

- 2 cups olive oil
- 12 each skewers
- ½ cup chopped fresh parsley
- 4 lb. large shrimp, peeled and deveined with tails attached
- 2 lemon, juiced
- 2 tsp. ground black pepper
- 2 tsp. salt
- 1 tbsp. dried oregano
- 2 tbsp. tomato paste
- 6 garlic cloves, minced
- ¼ cup hot pepper sauce

DIRECTIONS

1. In a mixing bowl, stir together parsley, oregano, olive oil, hot sauce, garlic, lemon juice, tomato paste, salt, and black pepper. Reserve a small amount to use later.

2. Pour remaining marinade into a large resealable plastic bag with shrimp. Seal, and marinate in the refrigerator for a couple of hours.

3. Preheat grill for medium-low heat. Thread shrimp onto skewers, then discard marinade.

4. Lightly oil grill grate. Cook shrimp for 4/5 minutes per side, basting frequently with reserved marinade.

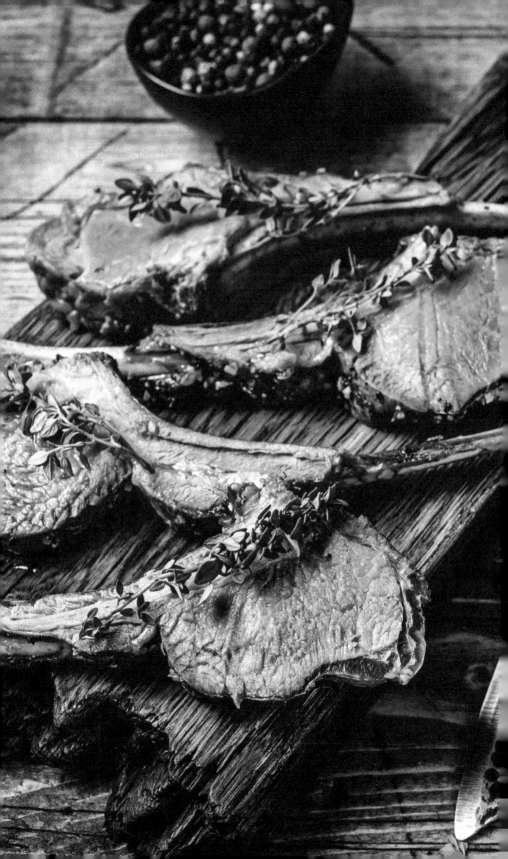

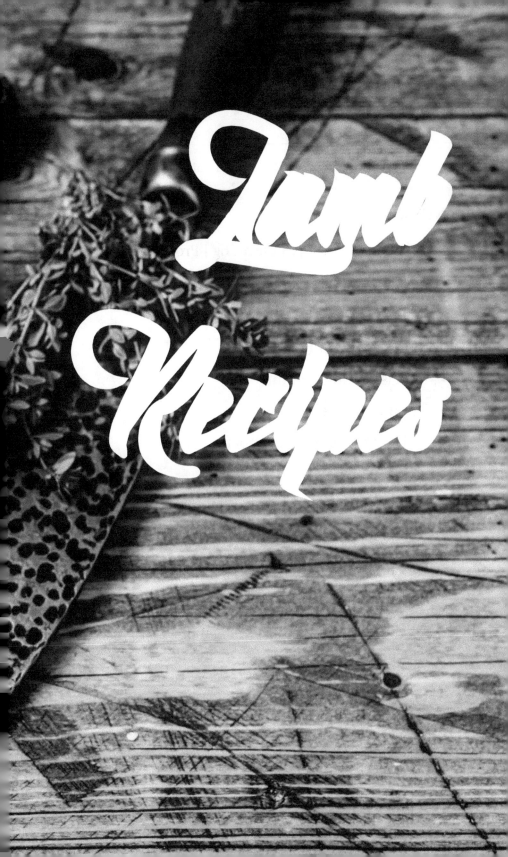

Lamb Recipes

GRILLED LAMB BURGER

Prep. Time: 10 min	Cook Time: 15 min	Servings:8

NUTRITION

Calories: 341 | Fat: 24g | Carbs: 6g | Protein: 21g.

INGREDIENTS

- 2 lb. lean ground lamb
- 2 dash ground cumin
- 1 onion, grated
- 1 tsp. ground black pepper
- 1 tsp. salt
- 4 garlic cloves, pressed
- 1 tsp. ground coriander
- 1 tsp. dried savory
- 1 tsp. ground allspice
- 2 slice bread, toasted and crumbled

DIRECTIONS

1. Preheat an outdoor grill for medium-high heat, and lightly oil grate.

2. In large bowl, combine ground lamb, garlic, onion, and breadcrumbs. Season with cumin, coriander, salt, pepper.

3. Knead until mixture is stiff. Shape into 8 very thin patties.

4. Cook patties for about 6 minutes on each side, or until cooked through.

AMAZING LAMB KABOBS

Prep. Time: 25 min	Cook Time: 13 min	Servings:10

INGREDIENTS

- 2½ lb. boneless lamb shoulder, cut into 1-inch pieces
- 2 tbsp. melted butter
- 3 tbsp. mustard
- ½ (10-oz.) jar maraschino cherries, drained and juice reserved
- 2 onions, quartered
- 2 tbsp. white wine vinegar
- 2 tbsp. olive oil
- 1 tbsp. cherry tomatoes
- Salt and black pepper, to taste
- ¼ tsp. crumbled dried sage
- ¼ tsp. chopped fresh rosemary
- 2 garlic cloves, chopped
- ½ (16-oz.) can pineapple chunks, drained with juice reserved
- 2 green bell peppers, cut into large chunks
- ½ (10-oz.) package whole fresh mushrooms

DIRECTIONS

1. Place lamb in a large bowl.

2. In a separate bowl, mix together olive oil, vinegar, mustard, salt, pepper, sage, rosemary, and garlic. Pour over lamb and mix to coat meat.

3. Cover, and refrigerate overnight.

4. Preheat outdoor grill for direct heat.

5. Add marinated fruit, lamb, and vegetables to skewers. Reserve some of the juice from cherries and pineapple chunks.

6. Mix together in a small bowl, melted butter and splashes of juice from the pineapples and cherries to create a basting sauce.

7. Place skewers on preheated grill, and cook about 13 minutes, turning and brushing with butter sauce.

NUTRITION

Calories: 398 | Fat: 29g | Carbs: 14g | Protein: 21g.

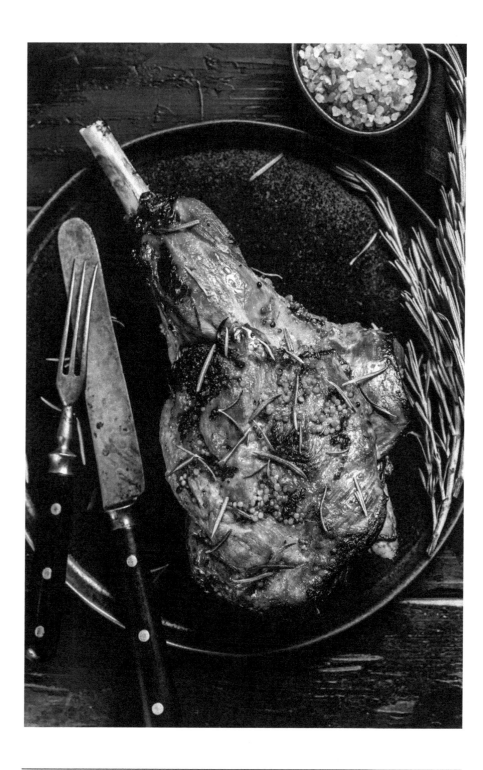

GRILLED LAMB LEG

Prep. Time: 15 min	Cook Time: 10 min	Servings:6

NUTRITION

Calories: 332 | Fat: 22g | Carbs: 2g | Protein: 31g.

INGREDIENTS

- 6 bone-in lamb steaks
- Salt and ground black pepper, to taste
- ⅓ cup olive oil
- 1 tbsp. chopped fresh rosemary
- 6 large garlic cloves, minced

DIRECTIONS

1. Put lamb steaks in a single layer in a shallow dish. Cover with rosemary, garlic, olive oil, salt, and pepper. Flip steaks to coat both sides. Let sit until steaks absorb flavors, about half an hour.

2. Preheat an outdoor grill for high heat and lightly oil the grate. Cook steaks until browned on the outside and slightly pink in the center, about 4-5 minutes per side for medium (ideal temperature 140°F)

EASY GRILLED LAMB CHOPS

Prep. Time: 10 min	Cook Time: 7 min	Servings:12

NUTRITION

Calories: 520 | Fat: 42g | Carbs: 3g | Protein: 26g.

INGREDIENTS

- ½ cup distilled white vinegar
- 2 tbsp. minced garlic
- 4 lb. lamb chops
- 2 onion, thinly sliced
- 1 tbsp. salt
- 1 tsp. black pepper
- ¼ cup olive oil

DIRECTIONS

1. Stir together garlic, vinegar, onion, salt, pepper, and olive oil in a large resealable bag until the salt has dissolved. Add lamb, toss until coated, and marinate in refrigerator for a couple of hours.

2. Preheat an outdoor grill for medium-high heat.

3. Remove lamb from the marinade and leave any onions on that stick to the meat. Discard any remaining marinade. Wrap the exposed ends of the bones with aluminum foil to keep them from burning.

4. Grill to desired doneness, about 3 minutes per side for medium.

HERBED LAMB CHOPS

Prep. Time: 25 min	Cook Time: 10 min	Servings:8

NUTRITION

Calories: 558 | Fat: 49g | Carbs: 6g | Protein: 16g.

INGREDIENTS

- 1 cup olive oil
- 8 lamb chops
- 1 cup balsamic vinegar
- 2 tsp. black pepper
- 2 tsp. chopped fresh parsley
- 2 tsp. dried tarragon
- ½ cup white wine
- 4 garlic cloves, peeled and minced
- ¼ cup lemon juice
- ½ cup minced onion

DIRECTIONS

1. In a large container blend the olive oil, white wine, vinegar, garlic, lemon juice, and onion. Season with parsley, tarragon, and pepper. Place lamb chops in the mixture. Cover, and marinate in the refrigerator about a couple of hours.

2. Preheat an outdoor grill for high heat, and lightly oil grate.

3. Grill lamb chops on the prepared grill about 5 minutes per side (ideal temperature of 145°F). Discard remaining marinade.

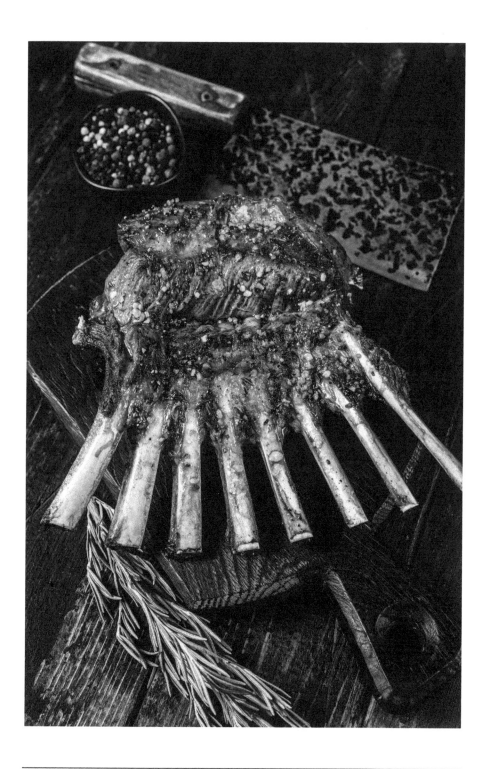

CPSIA information can be obtained
at www.ICGtesting.com
Printed in the USA
LVHW080144200821
695726LV00002B/69